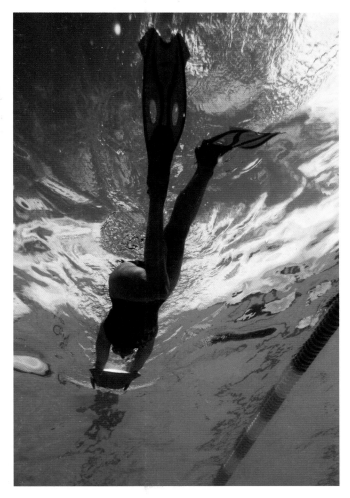

SWIMMING
FOR EXERCISE

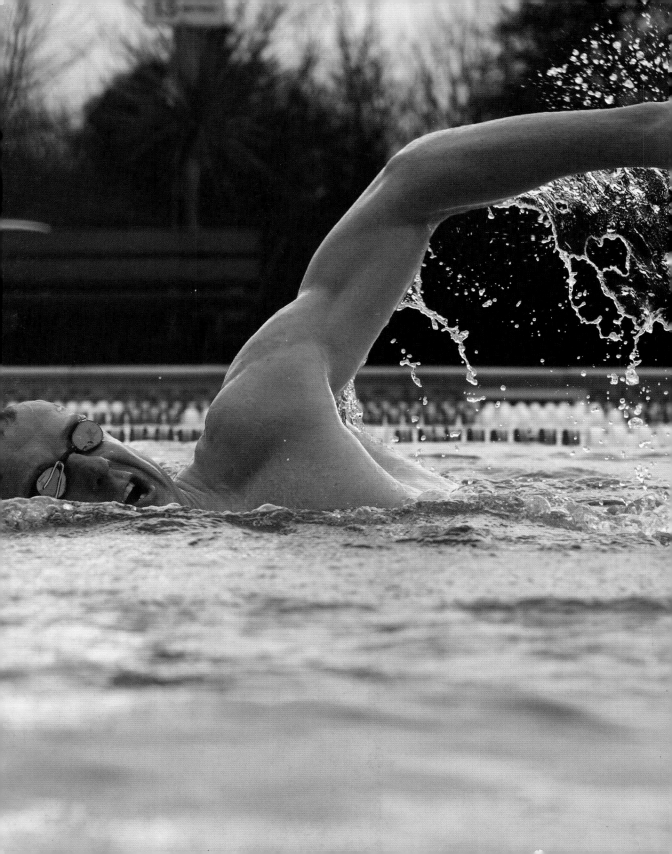

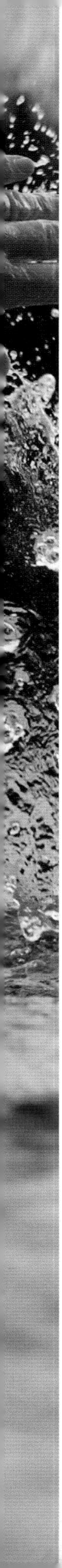

SWIMMING
FOR EXERCISE

OPTIMIZE YOUR TECHNIQUE, FITNESS AND ENJOYMENT

Greg Whyte

Photography by Eddie Jacob

FIREFLY BOOKS

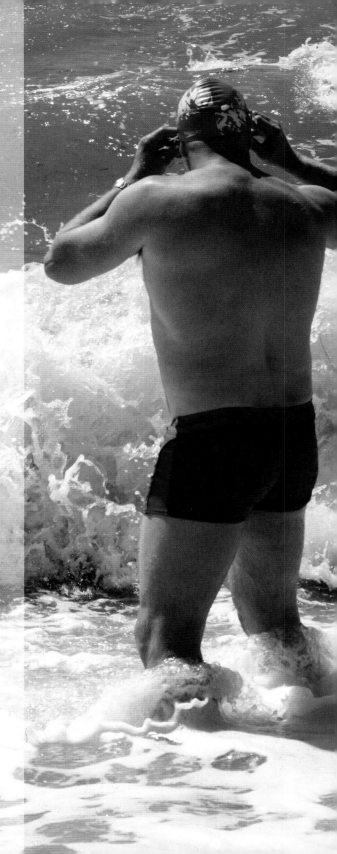

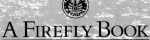

A FIREFLY BOOK

Published by Firefly Books Ltd. 2011

First printing

Publisher Cataloging-in-Publication Data (U.S.)

Whyte, Greg.
   Swimming for exercise : optimize your technique, fitness and enjoyment / Greg Whyte.
[144] p. : col. photos. ;   cm.
Includes index.
Summary: A handbook designed to improve technique and performance in the water.
ISBN-13: 978-1-55407-822-6 (pbk.)
ISBN-10:1-55407-822-9 (pbk.)
1. Swimming. 2. Exercise.   I. Title.
797.21 dc22   GV837.W598 2010

Library and Archives Canada Cataloguing in Publication

Whyte, Gregory P.
        Swimming for Exercise / Greg Whyte.
Includes Index.
ISBN-13: 978-1-55407-822-6
ISBN-10: 1-55407-822-9
        1. Swimming   I. Title
GV837.W59   2011   797.2'1
C2010-905850-X

Published in the United States by
Firefly Books (U.S.) Inc.
P.O. Box 1338, Ellicott Station
Buffalo, New York 14205

Published in Canada by
Firefly Books Ltd.
66 Leek Crescent
Richmond Hill, Ontario L4B 1H1

Cover design: Louise Leffler

Cover photography: Eddie Jacob

Printed in China

Developed by:
Kyle Cathie Limited

For Kyle Cathie:
Project editor: Jenny Wheatley
Designer: Louise Leffler
Photographer: Eddie Jacob
Copy editor: Anne Newman
Editorial assistant: Catharine Robertson
Production: Gemma John
Models: Rosie Edwards, Monjana Fyfe, Raquel Meseguer, Karen Pickering, Laura Wheatley, Greg Whyte, Steve Whyte, Maya Whyte, Elise Whyte, Mathew Wilson, and Ruby Wilson.

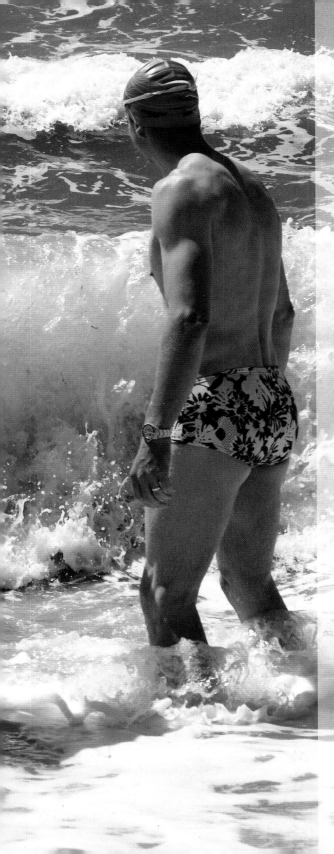

CONTENTS

· ·

FOREWORD

I met Greg at the 1992 Barcelona Olympics where we were both competing in our first Olympic Games. We remained friends during our competitive careers until Greg retired after the 1996 Atlanta Olympics—he is a bit older than me! Greg then moved into sport science where he became the Director of Research for the British Olympic Association and head of the Olympic acclimatization strategy for Team GB. As I was still competing I got to see Greg as a scientist at the 2000 and 2004 Olympic Games. The transition from world leading athlete to world leading scientist makes Greg a unique individual in the world of sports.

Following my retirement from international swimming I launched Karen Pickering SWIM and now have swim schools at venues across the UK for children and adults of all ages and abilities. As an Olympian, swimming has been my passion and an important part of my life for many years but, since establishing my swim schools, I now appreciate the key role swimming has to play in promoting an active and healthy lifestyle and how it can dramatically improve your quality of life. It is the only sport that can be enjoyed by all ages, shapes, and sizes and learning to swim could save your life. Now my passion is encouraging as many people as possible to take up the sport I love and still continue to enjoy so much today.

With his background in international sports and sports science Greg is uniquely placed to write *Swimming for Exercise*. Greg's experience as an international athlete and his status as one of the world's leading sports scientists means that *Swimming for Exercise* offers the reader a wonderfully visual, clear, and concise resource. It has everything you need to know about swimming, from getting started in the water to improving your technique and performance, as well as expanding your swimming horizons to competitive and open-water swimming. *Swimming for Exercise* is a must for everyone interested in swimming.

Karen Pickering

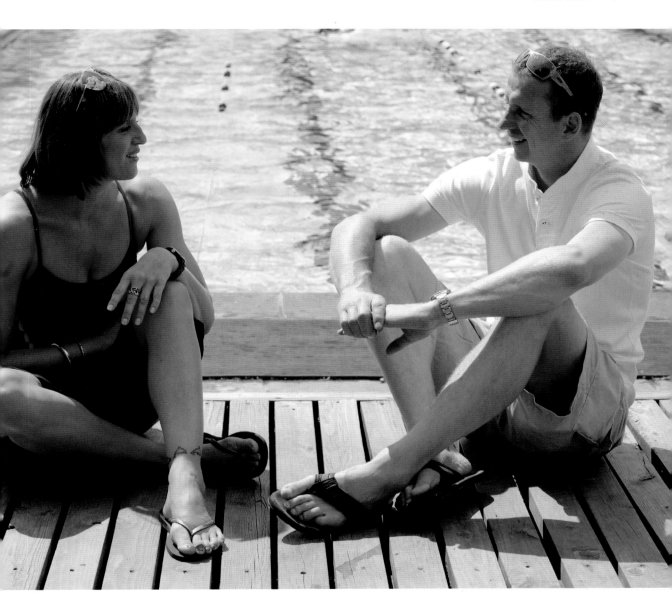

INTRODUCTION

Five-thirty a.m. on a cold, dark winter's morning. I am awoken by a tap, tap, tapping on my bedroom door and a voice whispering, "Time to get up for training, Greg." The voice is that of my dad, George, who was my coach during the formative part of my early sporting career and remained a mentor through the good times—and the bad—of a life spent in the water. Early-morning sessions, five times per week (plus five evenings), were the mainstay of my swimming training, and while the early-morning rise sometimes felt like a chore, I always felt invigorated as I sat down to a hearty breakfast, having finished my ninety-minute session as the rest of the world was just waking.

But swimming is not just for Olympians; in fact, for the vast majority of swimmers, it isn't even competitive. It is the most popular form of sporting activity, and is one of the few that can be enjoyed by both males and females of all ages, both with and without disabilities. Swimming plays an important part in tackling an array of physical and mental health problems and can help to reduce the incidence of over twenty chronic illnesses, including heart disease, diabetes, and cancer. It is also an excellent form of exercise for those carrying excess weight, including pregnant women.

In addition to pool swimming, the opportunity to experience incredible open-water swims is on the increase with the establishment of specialized swim-tour companies offering swimming experiences all over the world. When the triathlon emerged as a new sport, later on in my career, in the late 1990s, it was an absolute revelation. This exciting multi-event used all types of open water for the first leg of the race, from pools to lakes, rivers, and sea; it was still swimming, but it felt entirely different.

Despite having had a wonderful life as a competitive swimmer, it wasn't until I retired, in my late twenties, that I truly began to enjoy swimming. With competition no longer the sole reason for swimming, I was able to expand my horizons. I started to look at different bodies of water, wondering what it would be like to swim them. Deep lakes and seas, a long way from land, hold their own challenges: overcoming fears of deep water and what might lie beneath is an important step (swimming with others always helps calm the nerves) and coping with the changing elements, including the waves and saltwater, leads to an unparalleled sense of achievement.

In recent years, I have been incredibly fortunate to have been able to take on some of the world's most iconic swims, including the English Channel with David Walliams and the Gibraltar Straits with James Cracknell (and a pod of whales!). I have even swum from the UK to the U.S.! (In fact, it was the British Virgin Isles to the U.S. Virgin Isles in the Caribbean, somewhat shorter at 4 miles, but an incredible swim with some amazing wildlife!)

Having said all of this, while pool swimming can be tedious and seem fruitless at times, even for a competitive swimmer, years of experience have taught me ways to enhance it, while optimizing fitness and performance gains. If you already swim, want to start swimming again after a long time out of the water, or are starting now for the first time, this book will provide you with all the advice and information you will need to fully enjoy swimming.

Greg Whyte

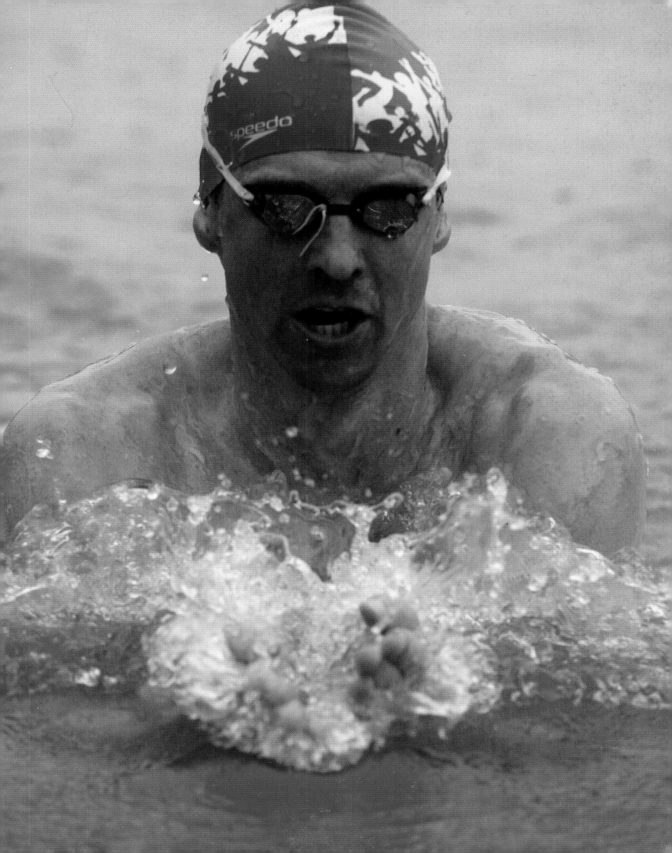

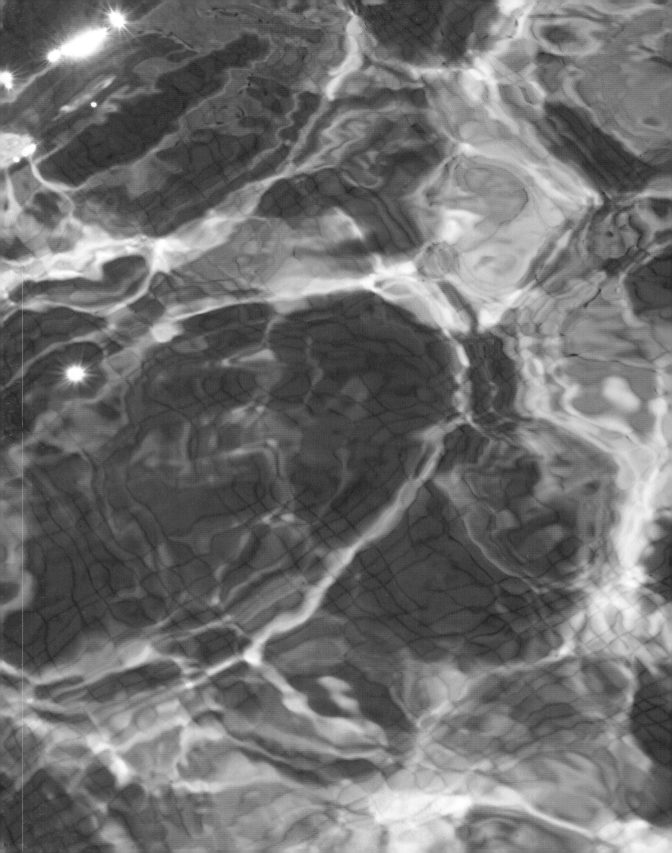

chapter 1

What's so great about swimming?

THE BENEFITS

Swimming can be enjoyed all year round and is a great form of exercise for everyone. You can swim in a safe, controlled environment, alone or with friends, from early morning to late at night. Unlike many other forms of exercise, you don't have to be at the same level as your friends to be able to enjoy it together; you can choose your own stroke and pace and comfortably share the pool with anyone. The warm waters of the swimming pool are comforting and therapeutic, and because the water supports your body weight, it is not a problem if you are carrying a couple of extra pounds. In the same way, it is a great form of exercise during pregnancy, and is safe for expectant mothers all the way through to term—including delivery for those choosing the water-birth option! The warm water and reduced joint stress also make swimming ideal for those suffering from joint problems like arthritis.

As a whole-body exercise, swimming gives you a great workout and tones all of your muscles, thereby improving fitness levels. It also leads to improved health that can positively affect your physical, mental, social and spiritual well-being. Research has shown that increasing the amount of exercise you do and improving your fitness decreases the chance of developing a range of chronic diseases. In addition, swimming benefits your mind by improving mood, reducing anxiety and increasing self-confidence. So swimming works from head to toe, and from inside to outside, helping you to look great and feel even better.

In addition to the direct effects on health and well-being, swimming can increase the success of dieting. This is due to the fact that by exercising regularly you are more likely to maintain a healthy lifestyle overall, which in turn leads to higher self-esteem and increased self-confidence, something that dieting alone rarely achieves (only 10 percent of those who diet are able to maintain weight reduction in the long term).

Added to all this, swimming will give you that "feel-good factor" and improve your quality of life. In other words, it will add life to your years as well as years to your life.

How much swimming should I do?

The message is simple: anything is better than nothing! The World Health Organization suggests that 150 minutes of exercise per week is needed for health. But you don't have to start with 150 minutes or do that amount all in one go; you can accumulate it in shorter, more targeted sessions. In my experience, gradually increasing the amount of time you spend exercising over weeks and months is much more successful than an instant dramatic increase in your exercise program.

You can make swimming your predominant form of exercise or intergrate it into your weekly regime to add variety and a change of environment. Because we are all different, it is important that you tailor your program to your own individual needs, organizing it into manageable and enjoyable chunks. That way, you will get the most out of your swimming, reach your goals more easily and learn new skills. Altogether swimming can prolong and improve the quality of your life. Formulating a program that works for you will increase your enjoyment and help you to maintain your swimming in the long term.

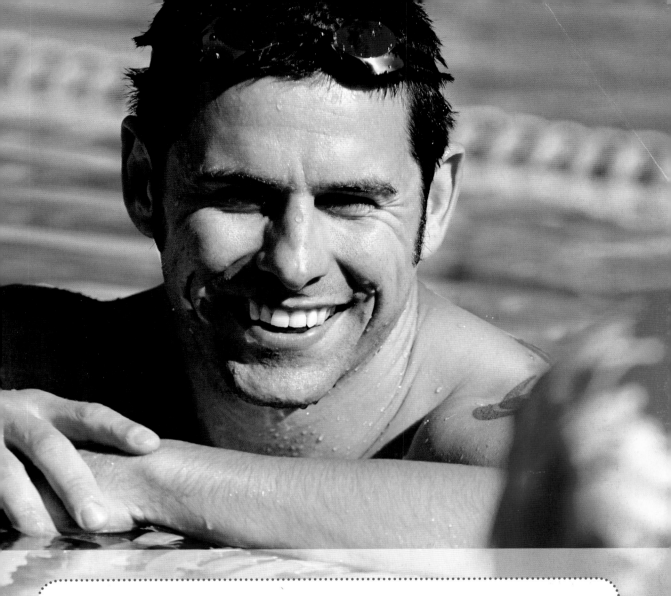

SWIMMING: GOOD FOR YOUR MIND, BODY, AND SOUL

Increased levels of physical activity and fitness are linked to a reduction in the development of over twenty chronic diseases including heart disease, stroke, diabetes, and cancer. Swimming is a great form of exercise and has a number of important psychological benefits, not least improved mood, reduced anxiety, and increased self-confidence. In addition to the direct effects on health and well-being, exercise leads to a better all-around lifestyle and puts you in a better position to succeed with dieting and stopping smoking, should you need to do so.

GETTING STARTED

Unlike most forms of exercise, swimming is potentially quite dangerous if you have never done it before! There are a large number of people who can't swim because they have never had the opportunity, or because they are so afraid of water that they have not tried it before. There are also people who can swim very short distances, but lack the confidence to go swimming alone. Swimming lessons are a great option for anyone who fits into these categories. All local pools run classes for all ages and abilities. Confidence is a crucial part of learning to swim, and having expert guidance while swimming alongside other newcomers is the best way to build it. Don't be afraid to sign up for swimming lessons; you will be surprised how popular they are and how many other people can't swim. Simply go to your local rec center or health club and ask for details. Alternatively, search for local swimming lessons on the internet.

Fit to swim?

If you are returning to swimming after a long absence from the water, it is important that you start your program slowly and build it up gradually. Don't think you can just pick up where you left off—unfortunately, fitness gains are quickly lost if you have not swum for a long period, so you may find your fitness is not as good as you remember it! Having said that, swimming is like riding a bike in that although your technique might become a little rusty, you never forget it, and within a couple of sessions you will quickly get back into the swing of it. Importantly, if you haven't exercised for a long time, you should treat yourself as a first-time exerciser and take the usual health precautions before starting a program (see page 16).

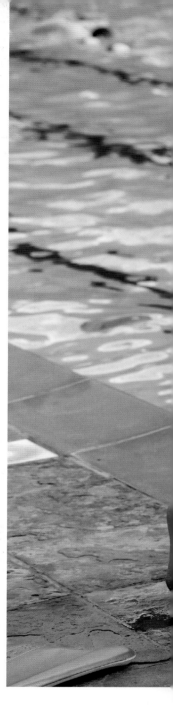

RIGHT: Expert help—getting the help of a coach can be the shortcut to technical excellence.

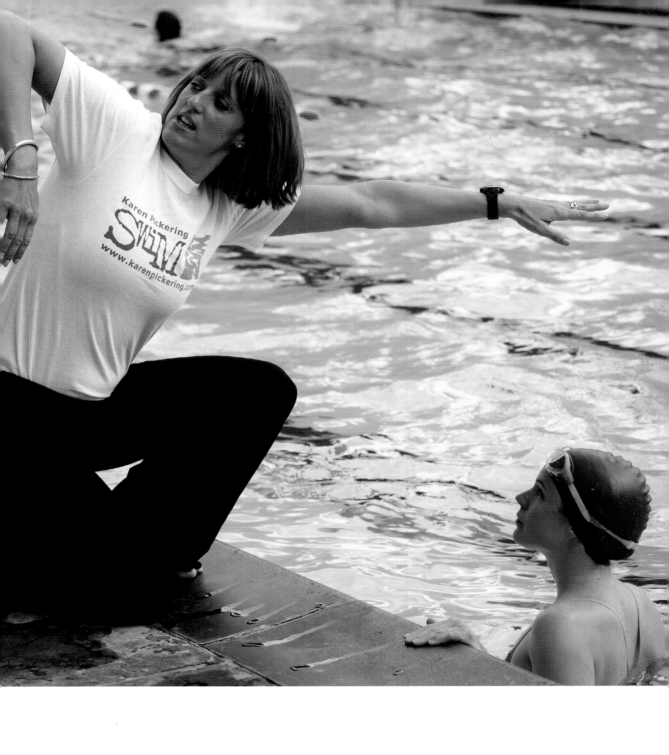

GET THE GO-AHEAD TO SWIM

Because of the increased stress placed upon the body, particularly the cardiovascular and pulmonary systems (heart, blood vessels, and lungs), swimming does carry some risks for those individuals with preexisting disease. Sometimes it is not always obvious if you have a disease that may be affected by exercise; coronary heart disease, for example, may only be noticeable when you start to exercise and place the heart under increased stress. If you answer "Yes" to any of the following questions, consult your doctor before starting a swimming program:

- Has your doctor ever told you that you have a heart condition?

- Do you feel pain in your chest during physical activity?

- Have you recently suffered from chest pain at rest?

- Do you suffer from dizziness?

- Have you ever lost consciousness?

- Do you suffer from joint problems that may be made worse by exercise?

- Are you currently taking drugs for high blood pressure, high cholesterol, or a heart condition?

- Do you know of any reason why you should not participate in exercise?

You should also contact your doctor before starting swimming if:

- You already have a diagnosed chronic health problem (including heart or lung disease and diabetes) or are at high risk of developing one.

- You are over the age of forty and inactive.

RIGHT: The ease of swimming—all you need is a swimsuit, a towel, and goggles to get started.

Swimming for health

Despite the need to highlight the necessary precautions you should take if you feel you are at risk, it is important to remember that exercise plays an important role in both managing and treating health problems. Even if you have chronic disease, exercise is rarely discouraged altogether. In fact, it is often promoted by the medical community in such circumstances, the only difference being that somewhat more caution is recommended. Unfortunately, in my experience, it is often those with chronic disease who feel least able to exercise for fear of the possible difficulties, even though they are often the ones who stand to gain the most from it. A careful approach in close consultation with the medical community and a personal trainer is the best way to help to allay fears while promoting an active lifestyle. This is the same advice I give those starting exercise for the first time or returning to exercise after a long period of inactivity.

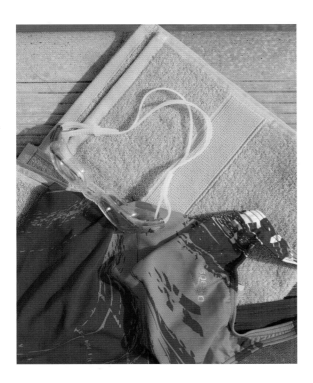

What gear do I need?

Swimming is relatively simple when it comes to equipment—all you really need is a swimsuit. Of course, as with most sporting pastimes, there is a wealth of paraphernalia that accompanies swimming (see Gadgets and Gizmos, page 74), but the most important additions are goggles and a towel. This simplicity is probably what makes swimming so popular.

Choosing the right swimsuit is important for comfort and performance, as well as fashion! While the choice of suits for men is relatively simple (briefs, trunks or board-shorts), for women there is a range of styles available from one-piece suits with various shapes around the shoulders (e.g. racerback, powerback, crossback, leaderback), to the many bikini options. Deciding on the right swimsuit for you is often a case of trial and error, but you can obtain some general guidance from your local sportswear store or on various swimming manufacturers' websites (see Resources, page 140).

How much swimming should I do at the start?

To avoid injury and soreness, start off with just a small amount of easy swimming, then gradually build on this over time. "Swimming volume" is a term used to describe how much you swim, taking into account how long you swim for, how hard you swim, and how often you swim. You can monitor your swimming volume to ensure that you are progressing at a rate that suits you. It is best to avoid massive increases in swimming volume over short periods of time—even for the experienced swimmer, rapid increases in volume can lead to injury and illness. The distance and speed you swim should be challenging but achievable to reduce the possibility of problems and optimize your enjoyment.

What do I do once I'm in the pool?

Swimmers are a regimented lot, and in general there is strict etiquette when it comes to lane swimming. In most pools each lane has a designated direction and speed, and it is important both for the safety and enjoyment of all concerned that you observe the direction of swimming in the lane. You must also select the lane speed that is appropriate to you; apart from annoying other swimmers if you are swimming too slowly (or too fast) for your lane, you will reduce your enjoyment if you are continually being overtaken or are trying to overtake. Finding the correct lane is usually a case of trial and error, but the best policy is to start in a slower lane and move up rather than get swamped by the faster swimmers.

If you are just starting to swim or returning after a long period out of the water, you may wish to swim where there is more freedom to stop and start when needed without being constrained by lengths and ropes. The best thing for newcomers is to use the free space next to the lanes or to swim when there are no lanes in place and you are able to swim widths instead of lengths. This means you can also stay close to the wall in shallower water where you can touch the sides or bottom if you need to. Remember, swimming is about confidence; don't push yourself too hard too fast.

When should I swim?

The great thing about swimming is you can swim any time of day, seven days a week, 365 days of the year, and in any weather. Even on those dark, cold winter nights when you don't want to go outside, the pool is warm and bright.

Swimming is great exercise at any time of day, but particularly so in the early morning. At this time of day, when other load-bearing forms of exercise like running seem far too hard on the body, the warmth and support of the pool makes swimming a much more inviting option.

There are only very few occasions when you shouldn't swim. Take care not to swim too soon after eating a large meal—cramps are common when swimming after eating and the last thing you want is to be in the water and unable to continue swimming. It is wise to leave one to two hours between a big meal and a swim. Also, never swim after consuming alcohol as it can impair your judgment, encourage risk-taking behavior, reduce your coordination and reaction time, and lead to early fatigue and confusion. Swimming while under the influence of alcohol can be dangerous and life-threatening both to yourself and to others.

For women, there is no reason why you can't swim at any time during your menstrual cycle. In fact, exercise can often reduce the pain associated with menstruation and improve your overall mood, so keep on swimming!

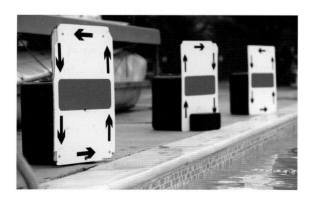

LEFT: Way to go—selecting the right lane to suit your own ability and swimming in the direction of the arrows will optimize your swimming experience.

SWIMMING IS FOR EVERYONE —SO NO EXCUSES!

It's easy to find reasons not to do something, but swimming really is something we can all do. Here are some of the most common excuses people use ... and the arguments against them.

"I'm too big to swim"

When you are carrying a couple of extra pounds most forms of exercise, particularly weight-bearing exercise like walking or jogging, can be too difficult or painful. Swimming, on the other hand, is not weight-bearing because the water supports the body weight. This means that there is no excess pressure on the joints, and you can enjoy a pain-free and effective workout. Also, because swimming is so technically demanding, it is often the case that the less proficient you are, the more energy you will expend traveling very small distances. In other words, the poorer your technique, the more energy you burn and the more weight you lose. At last, an activity you don't have to be good at to lose weight!

"Swimsuits are too revealing"

One of the main barriers to exercise when you are a little overweight is the way in which you think others view you, particularly in the gym or when out walking or jogging. Swimming creates a wonderfully safe environment in this respect—everyone is wearing a swimsuit and apart from the short walk from the changing room to the pool, you are submerged in water the whole time, where no one can really see you.

"I've got a bad back"

Over 80 percent of people in the United States will suffer from back pain at some time during their lives. Aside from the practical implications of this (for example, the many days lost from work), the most profound consequence of back pain is a reduced quality of life. If you suffer from back pain, swimming may be the ideal choice of exercise because it reduces the load bearing on your back, making it a more enjoyable form of exercise than many others. You will probably find that regular swimming helps to relieve back pain and can be effective in reducing its recurrence.

"I've got arthritis"

Osteoarthritis is the most common form of arthritis and the most prevalent disorder of the joints in middle-aged and older people, affecting the hands, hips, shoulders, and knees. Pain is often increased when the affected joint is used, particularly during load-bearing exercise. Swimming, however, reduces load bearing and, together with the warm water, helps reduce the pain of exercise, while protecting the joints and maintaining mobility. That's what makes swimming the exercise of choice for those with arthritis.

"I'm too old"

You are never too old to swim—the enormous health gains that swimming offers are available to everyone, irrespective of age. The warmth, buoyancy, and support offered by the water make swimming a great form of exercise in later life. It is a wonderful activity for those physical complaints that are so common as you get older, including joint pain, decreased flexibility and strength, and osteoporosis (low bone mineral density). You may need to alter the amount of swimming you do as you get older, but that's easy to do because you can regulate how hard, how long, and how often you swim in order to optimize the benefits. So keep on swimming to enhance both your physical and mental health, and to help enable you to enjoy life for as long as possible.

"I'm not physically able"

Swimming is a fantastic form of rehabilitation for those who have a reduced physical capacity due to a stroke, surgery, accident, or injury. The buoyancy and support offered by the water together with an array of buoyancy aids make swimming a safe and enjoyable form of exercise that can help physical development even for those with the most limited physical ability. And in addition to the physical benefits, the psychological benefits of this are enormous.

"I'm pregnant"

Swimming is fantastic for expectant mothers. The water supports the body and removes the load-bearing element common to other forms of exercise. This is particularly true for the pelvic floor. Because it is easy to self-regulate how long and how hard you swim, it is safe to do so through all three trimesters, right up to the birth. However, because of the increased laxity of the joints (increased range of motion) associated with hormonal changes in pregnancy, it is best to avoid the breast stroke in the third trimester.

The benefits of exercise during pregnancy include a reduction in gestational diabetes, pre-eclampsia, varicose veins, and constipation. Women who exercise during pregnancy have higher energy levels and happier pregnancies. But don't overdo it! Three to four thirty-minute swims per week is the sort of level to aim for, but it does depend on whether you were swimming before you were pregnant and your current level of conditioning. If you didn't exercise or only exercised a very small amount before getting pregnant, be realistic—a couple of sessions per week may suffice. If you were very active, you can swim more; just make sure that you are doing well with how much you are swimming.

OPPOSITE: Swimming is a great form of exercise during pregnancy.

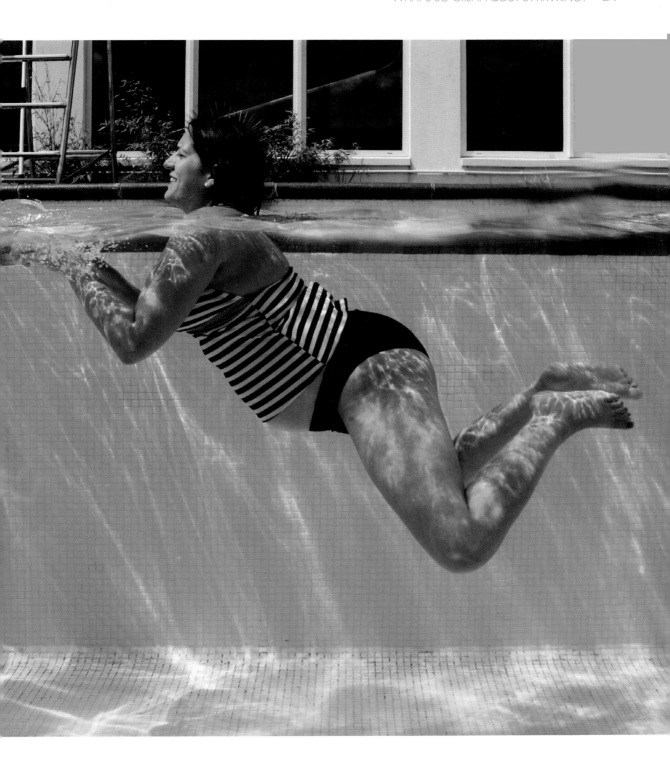

"My children are too young for swimming"

Kids instinctively love water, and encouraging your children to swim gives them a fantastic opportunity to develop a healthy and vibrant lifestyle. In addition, swimming is also a life skill that is potentially life-saving, whether their own or others'. Children can start swimming from a very early age, and often lessons start for babies as young as three months. However, general recommendations are for babies to have their third course of immunizations (usually at around sixteen weeks) prior to starting swimming.

So don't use your children as an excuse not to swim; rather, use them as a reason to swim. Sharing the adventure of swimming with your children is a good way to work out, increase confidence—yours and theirs—and have fun.

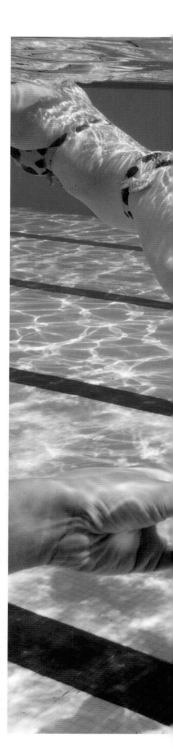

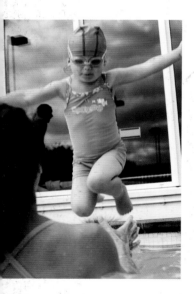

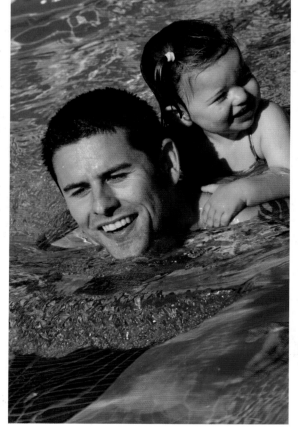

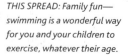

THIS SPREAD: Family fun— swimming is a wonderful way for you and your children to exercise, whatever their age.

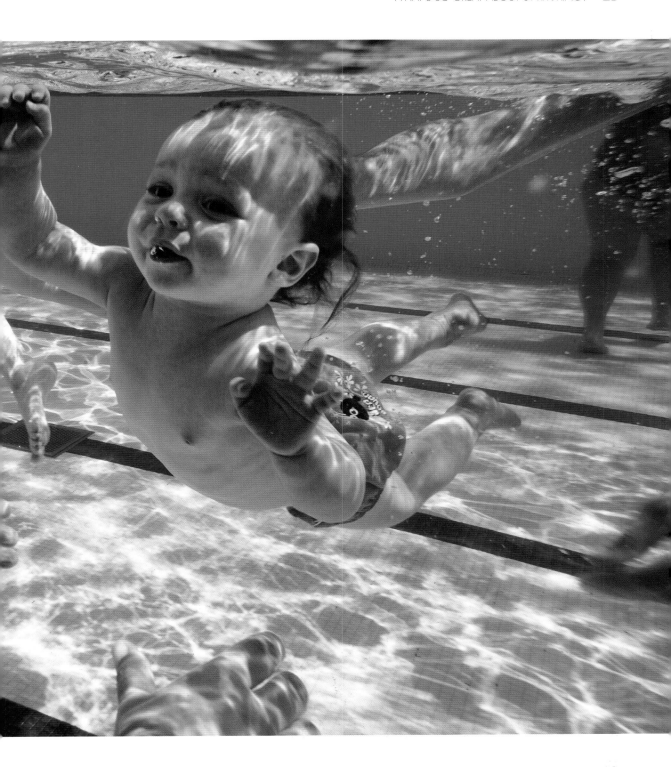

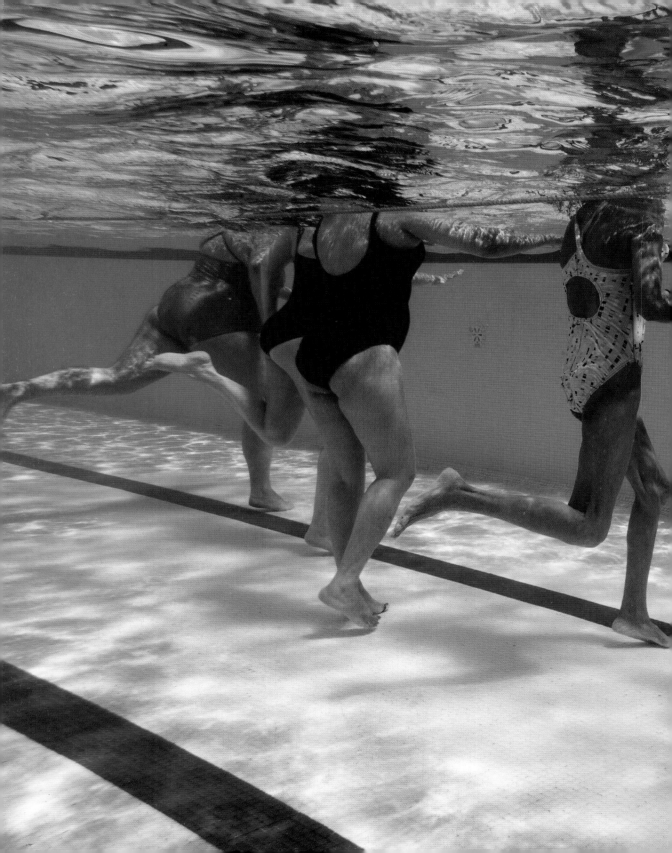

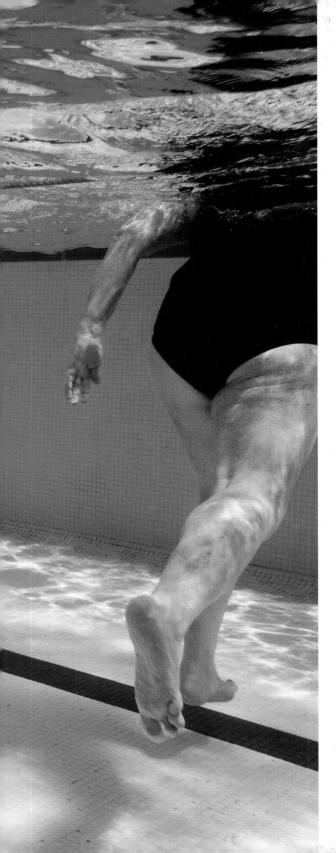

"I don't like swimming up and down in straight lines"

Enjoying the water is not all about lane swimming. Indeed, swimming up and down along the same black line every time you get in the water can become very tiresome. But there are lots of ways to work out in the pool without doing a single stroke. Aquarobics (basically aerobics in water, also known as aqua aerobics or water aerobics) is a fantastically fun way either to get fit or maintain fitness in the water. You don't even have to be able to swim to do it, and the buoyancy offered by the water can reduce the stresses and strains on your joints encountered on land. Despite taking away the impact, aquarobics increases the amount of energy you burn because you have to move through the increased resistance of water. So in a session of aquarobics you could burn 30–40 percent more calories than you would doing the same exercise on land! Plus, if you are a little self-conscious about your appearance, you can be completely invisible underwater.

Aquarobics is also perfect if you are injured or have joint problems. As well as reducing the impact, the warm waters of the pool can help to ease those aches and pains, making exercise a much more pleasant experience.

If you can't swim, aquarobics is a great way to increase your water confidence while getting fit at the same time; and if you can swim, but simply want a change, aquarobics is for you. As with any form of exercise, working out in a class can be highly motivating and great fun, so check out your local pool schedule, sign up for a class and enjoy!

LEFT: Be invisible—aquarobics is a great way to exercise whatever your shape or size.

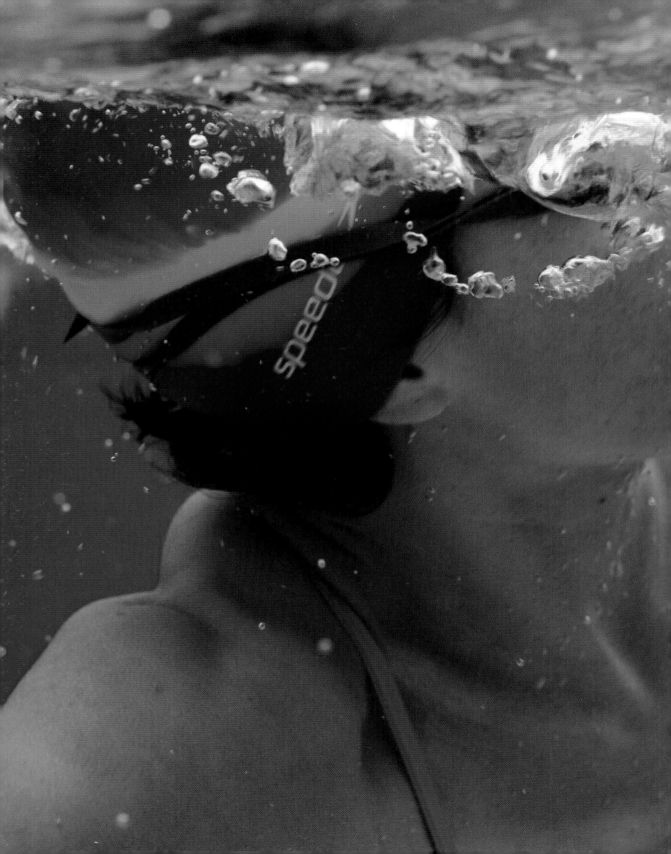

chapter 2

How to swim

THE FOUR STROKES

Most people have a favorite stroke, but being able to mix and match different strokes will enable you to make the most out of your time in the pool by offering you a more rounded workout and maximizing your enjoyment.

This chapter examines the technical aspects of the four major strokes, which are:

- front crawl
- breast stroke
- back stroke
- butterfly

The following technical guidelines and tips will help you improve your proficiency and style, and thus enhance your enjoyment of swimming. I have broken down the technique for each stroke into arms, kick and breathing, with each section describing the basics of the technique for optimal performance.

Swimming is highly technical and, as you will see, breaking the strokes down into precise movements of the arms and legs and then understanding the coordination of those movements can be confusing! The main thing is to remember that making even the smallest of changes to your technique is worthwhile and can have a profound effect on your overall economy and speed, and also reduce fatigue.

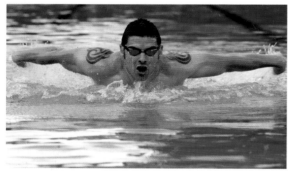

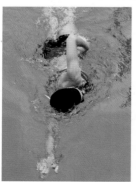

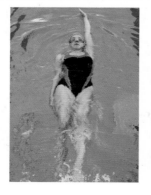

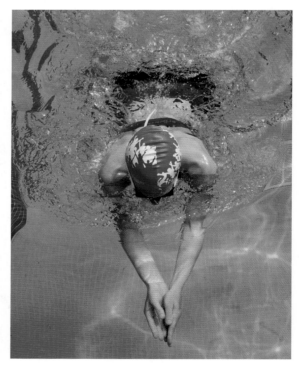

SWIMMING TERMINOLOGY

Entry
The entry of the hand into the water following the recovery (not applicable in breast stroke, as the hands remain underwater throughout).

Downsweep
When the hand moves down and away from the body prior to the catch phase (front crawl and back stroke are the only strokes to have a downsweep).

Outsweep
When the arms move away from the center line of the body at the start of the stroke (breast stroke is the only stroke to have an outsweep).

Catch Phase
The set-up for the propulsive phase of the stroke when the hands feel the pressure of the water.

Insweep
When the hands move toward the center line of the body in the middle of the stroke (front crawl, breast stroke, and butterfly all have an insweep).

Upsweep
When the hand moves up toward the surface of the water at the end of the stroke (front crawl, back stroke, and butterfly all have an upsweep).

Release
When the hand no longer feels the force of the water at the end of the stroke, just before it begins the recovery.

Recovery
The return of the arms to the starting point of the stroke (for front crawl, back stroke, and butterfly the recovery is above the water and for breast stroke it is under the water).

Flutter Kick
When the legs kick alternately (front crawl and back stroke use the flutter kick).

Glide
When the body is stretched out as long as possible and moving through the water with very little movement.

FRONT CRAWL

Front crawl uses an alternating arm stroke and a flutter kick (where the legs kick one at a time in a rhythmic fashion). Front crawl is the fastest stroke, and fairly easy to master. One stroke cycle consists of a right- and left-arm stroke and a varying number of kicks, dependent on the kick rhythm used. Throughout the stroke cycle, imagine you are on a rotisserie with a skewer through the center of your body: allow your body to roll from side to side along the central line.

The arms

The arm stroke consists of the following elements:

- Entry and stretch
- Downsweep and catch
- Insweep and upsweep
- Release and recovery

Entry and stretch

The arm enters the water fingertips first, followed by the hand and forearm. Entry of the arm is made in line with the shoulder, and your elbow should be slightly bent with your palm facing outward. The hand then pushes forward through the water, just below the surface, without crossing in front of the face (a common mistake is for the hand to swing across the body, distorting the body line). As you stretch your arm forward, turn your palm down **(see figure A)**.

Downsweep and catch

During this phase your arm flexes at the elbow and sweeps down. The catch begins when your hand is facing directly backward, your elbow is above your hand, and your forearm and upper arm are pushing backward against the water **(see figure B)**. At this point, your hand is slightly outside the line of your shoulder. This phase does not move you through the water, but merely serves to place the hand and arm in the correct position for the phase that moves you forward.

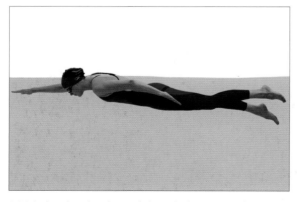

A Right hand pushes forward through the water in line with the right shoulder.

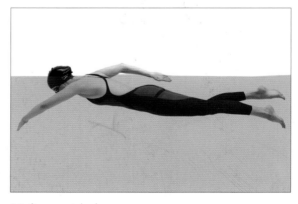

B Left arm catch phase.

Insweep and upsweep

The insweep begins just outside the line of the shoulder in the catch phase and finishes under the body in the midline. Your arm should be flexed at the elbow to around 90 degrees **(see figure C)**. From the end of the insweep, your arm extends slightly (not completely) and your palm pushes up toward your thigh. This is the upsweep—the most propulsive phase of the front crawl stroke where your hand is accelerating to its maximum speed. Think about your thumb touching your thigh as it approaches the surface of the water.

Release and recovery

During the recovery the elbow exits the water before the hand, and moves forward in a high arc **(see figure D)**. Because this phase is non-propulsive, try to expend as little energy as possible by keeping your arm relaxed. A common mistake is to allow the hand to lead the recovery, swinging it away from the body, which causes the body to wiggle.

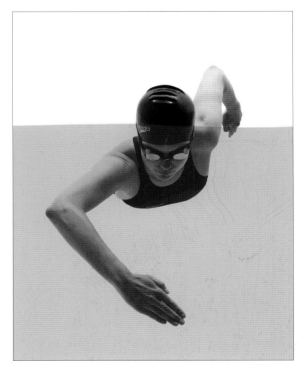

C Right arm insweep, elbow flexed to 90 degrees.

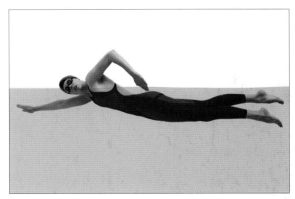

D The elbow exits the water before the hand.

Kicking

Front crawl uses the flutter kick, in which the legs kick alternately. Your kicking rhythm, i.e. the number of kicks per stroke cycle (usually two-beat, four-beat, or six-beat), will really depend on what works best for you.

Aim to kick from the hips and not the knees, and be sure to keep your ankles and feet relaxed and loose—as soon as you flex your feet the resistance causes your body to move in the opposite direction. The gap between your legs needs to be enough to offer your body stability without being too wide.

The commonest problem that I see is too much kicking with bent legs, which generates little forward propulsion and, in many cases, slows the swimmer down. Less is more when it comes to kicking for the recreational swimmer.

Breathing

Rhythmic and coordinated breathing is essential for efficient front crawl. Try not to lift your head out of the water when you breathe—instead, synchronize the rotation of your head with your arm movement and body roll. As your arm completes the upsweep and your body rolls toward it, turn your head as well, so that your mouth exits the water (see image opposite). You should find yourself breathing during the first half of the recovery phase and then rotating your head downward, back into the water, during the second half.

Avoid breathing every stroke and try to control your breathing by setting a rhythm. The commonest and most efficient rhythm is to breathe every three strokes, so that you take breaths on alternate sides. This is known as bilateral breathing and encourages good balance in the water.

TOP TIPS FOR FRONT CRAWL

- **Imagine you are swimming in a tube and try to keep all of your movements inside that tube.**

- **Relax your arm during the recovery and lead with the elbow (keeping the hand close to the body).**

- **Relax your kicking—overdoing it can be very tiring and make little difference in how fast you move.**

- **Breathe every third stroke, and avoid turning your head too much.**

- **Don't look down! Raise your eye line to look slightly in front of you—this will improve your body position.**

RIGHT: Everything in line and in sync—as the left arm starts the recovery, the body rolls to the left and the head rotates, allowing inhalation to occur.

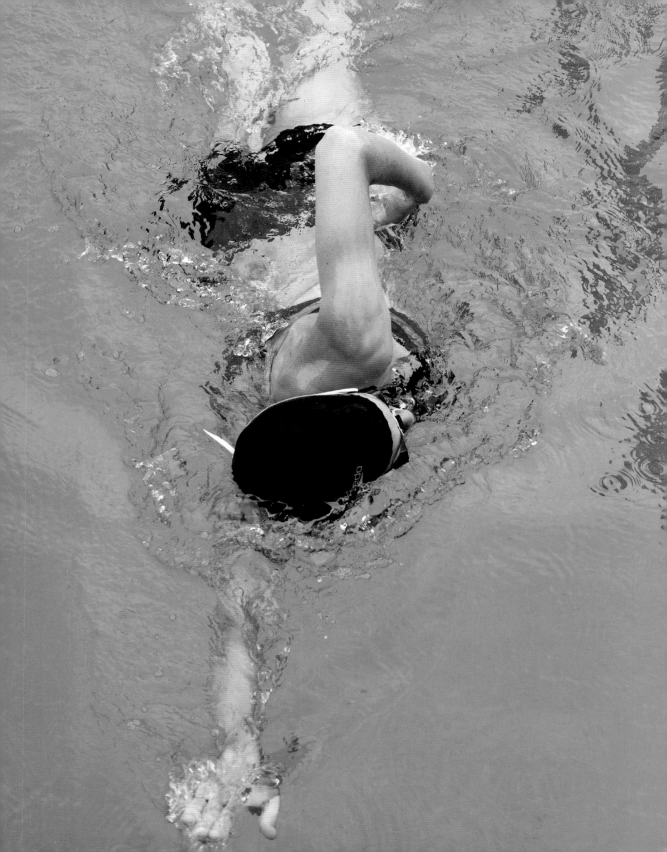

BREAST STROKE

Breast stroke is the slowest of the four strokes, and often the stroke of choice for the recreational swimmer because it is gentle and easy to master. That said, it is in fact the most technical stroke in terms of performance swimming.

The arms

The arm stroke consists of three elements:

- Outsweep
- Insweep
- Recovery

Outsweep
Your arms (with palms facing the bottom of the pool) sweep out to the catch phase **(see figure A)**. During the outsweep, your arms remain extended until just prior to the catch phase when they bend slightly. The outsweep is a slow, gentle action; a common mistake is to attack it with fast arms.

Insweep
This is the propulsive phase of the arm stroke, where your hands sweep in a semicircle downward and then upward motion until they are under the head with arms bent and elbows to the sides **(see figure B)**. Your hands accelerate gradually throughout the stroke.

Recovery
During the recovery you squeeze your elbows together so that your hands come under your chin **(see figure C)**. You then extend your arms forward to the glide position, with palms facing the bottom of the pool.

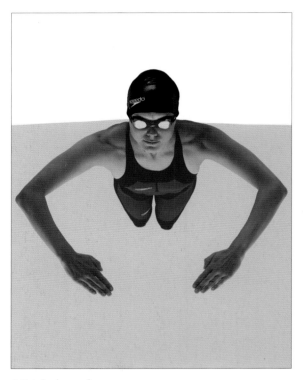

A Catch phase of arms.

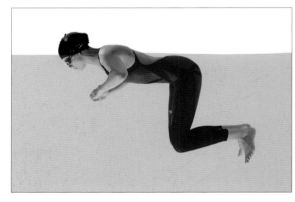

B Hands are under the head, knees are bent and shoulder-width apart.

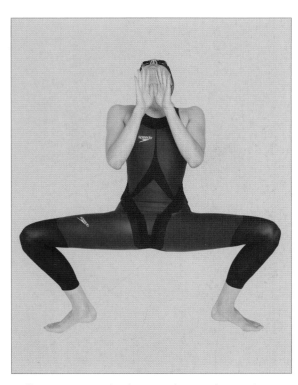

C Elbows come together, knees are bent, and toes point outward.

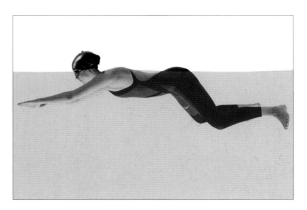

D Palms face the bottom of the pool, ankles are flexed.

Kicking

80 percent of the propulsion in breast stroke comes from the legs, which is why technique for the lower body is so important. The breast stroke leg kick is the most technically difficult element in swimming to execute correctly. It has three phases:

- Recovery
- Outsweep
- Insweep

Recovery

From the glide position (arms and legs extended) you bring your lower legs toward your bottom **(see figure B)**. A common mistake is to bring the knees toward the chest, which creates extra drag and slows you down, sometimes stopping you completely. Focus instead on bending at the knees and separate your legs slightly so that they are about shoulder-width apart.

Outsweep

As your feet reach your bottom, sweep your legs outward until they are outside the width of your hips, toes pointing outward and knees bent **(see figure C)**.

Insweep

Keeping your feet rotated outward extend your legs out, back, and down **(see figure D)**. The ankles should be flexed rather than floppy. At the end of the insweep the legs should be together and fully extended at the hips and the knees (glide position).

Coordination of the arms and legs

One breast stroke cycle consists of the arms stroking, followed by the legs kicking, and then a glide phase in which the arms and legs are fully extended. Timing is key in the breast stroke, and the coordination of the arms and legs can be broken down into three phases, as follows:

- the arms outsweep followed by the recovery of the legs;
- the arms insweep as the legs outsweep;
- the arms recover as the legs insweep.

To work on your timing you can extend the glide phase of the stroke and use it as a starting point for each cycle. Try it slowly at first, then speed up.

Breathing

For breast stroke you breathe once during each cycle. Correct breathing is crucial for the rhythm of the stroke; if you can get it right you will be on your way to a great technique.

Breathe out beneath the water during the glide phase, when you should be looking down at the bottom of the pool. Then, following the outsweep and insweep of the arms, lift your head as you squeeze your elbows together in the recovery. Your chin should be resting on the surface of the water, allowing you to inhale through your mouth (not your nose).

TOP TIPS FOR BREAST STROKE

- **Focus on the symmetry of your leg kick. A screw kick—when the legs are doing different things—is a common mistake.**

- **Don't pull your arms too wide— your elbows should never come past your shoulders. Imagine you are scooping the inside of a bowl rather than creating a huge sweeping circle.**

- **Keep your neck and shoulders relaxed and don't waste energy lifting your head up too high out of the water.**

- **Practice your technique slowly and only increase your speed once you have mastered the stroke.**

RIGHT: Timing is everything—as the arms extend forward in the recovery phase, the legs kick powerfully backward.

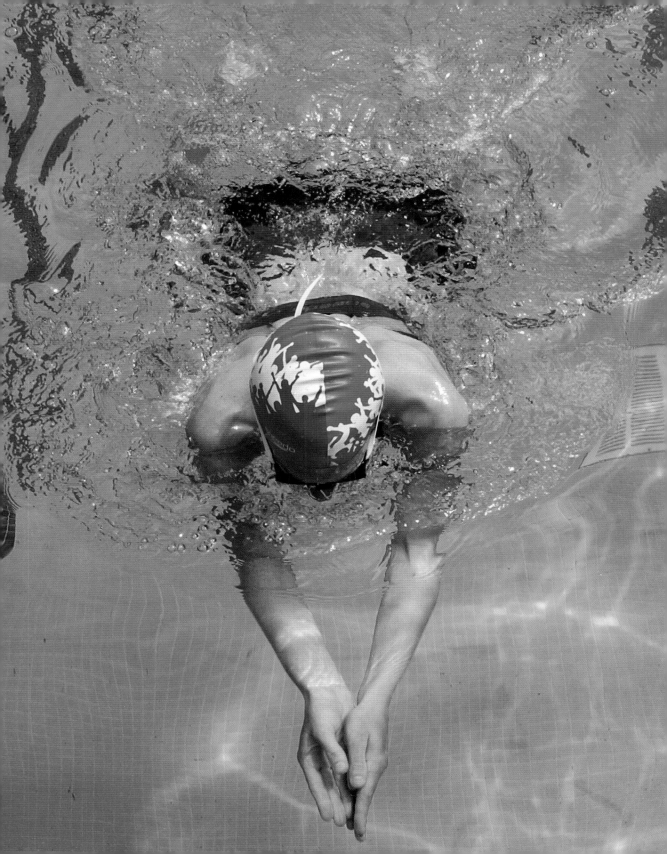

BACK STROKE

Back stroke tends to be the stroke least used by the recreational swimmer—perhaps due to the fact that it feels unnatural because you can't see where you are going! However, it is a great stroke for strengthening and toning the muscles without straining the back or neck.

Back stroke consists of an alternating arm stroke and a flutter kick. One stroke cycle consists of a right- and left-arm stroke with a continual leg kick. Throughout the stroke cycle you should imagine you are on a rotisserie with a skewer through the center of your body. Allow your body to roll from side to side along the central axis.

The arms

The arms provide the power in back stroke. The arm stroke consists of the following elements:

- Entry and downsweep
- Upsweep
- Release and recovery

Entry and downsweep

Your arm enters the water fully extended and directly in line with your shoulder. Your palm should be facing outward so that the little finger enters the water first **(see figure A)**. Following entry, sweep your arm down and out to the catch phase, in which the elbow is bent and the wrist is flexed **(see figure B)**.

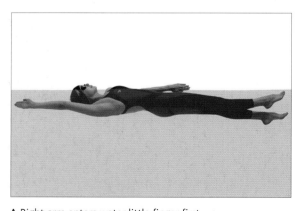

A Right arm enters water little finger first.

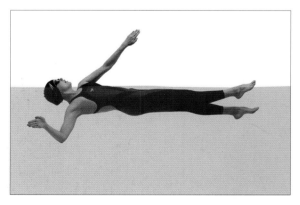

B Catch phase right arm.

Upsweep

From the catch phase push your hand toward your feet until the elbow is fully extended **(see figure C)**. At this point your arm will be below your thigh and your hand will be facing the bottom of the pool with your fingers facing the side.

Release and recovery

As your hand reaches the lower part of your thigh, relax it and turn the palm toward your body so that your thumb exits the water first. Lift your arm out of the water fully extended and move it in a pathway high and overhead. A common mistake is to swing the arms sideways, forcing the body to wiggle. During the recovery of the arm, rotate your wrist to enable your little finger to enter the water first **(see figure D)**.

Kicking

For back stroke the flutter kick is used, which is the same as the kick used in front crawl. Use a long, shallow kick initiated from the hips, not the knees. Try to keep the legs close together and your knees slightly bent, just under the surface of the water, throughout the kick. You should have floppy ankles and feet.

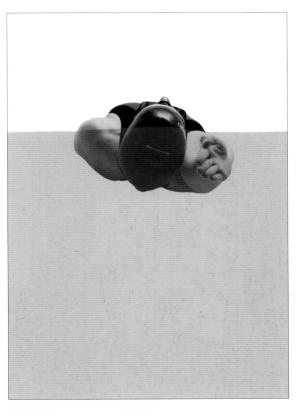

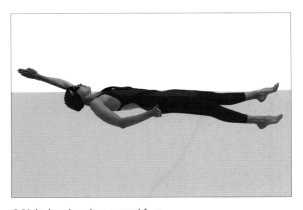

C Right hand pushes toward feet.

D Little finger enters water first.

Head position and breathing

A common mistake is to lift the head up and look toward the feet. This causes the hips to drop and creates extra resistance. Instead, look directly upward in order to maintain a flat body position near the surface of the water (this is a bit tougher when you swim outdoors!). Because the face is out of the water, breathing during back stroke is generally easier than for other strokes. However, it is nonetheless beneficial to create and maintain a breathing rhythm in order to support your stroke technique.

TOP TIPS FOR BACK STROKE

- **As with the front crawl, imagine you are swimming in a tube— try to keep all of your movements inside that tube.**

- **Do not let your hips drop too low—push them upward toward the ceiling to maintain a good body position.**

- **Allow your head to be fully supported by the water so that your neck can relax.**

- **Do not kick too much—kicking can be very tiring without making a big difference in how fast you move.**

- **Breathe consistently and evenly.**

RIGHT: No resistance—the body is stretched out as the left arm enters and the right arm exits the water.

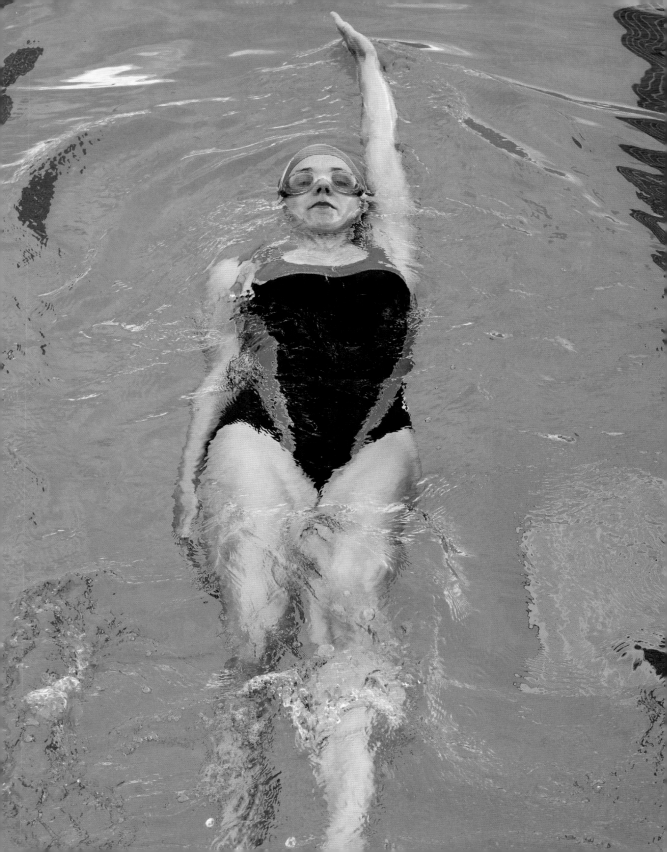

BUTTERFLY

Butterfly is widely considered to be the most demanding stroke, mainly because of the difficult coordination of the arms and legs, and also the shoulder strength required. One stroke cycle consists of the arms stroking together combined with two dolphin kicks.

The arms

The arm stroke consists of the following elements:

- Entry and catch
- Insweep and upsweep
- Release and recovery

Entry and catch

Your arms should enter the water at the same time, shoulder-width apart, palms facing outward **(see figure A)**. After entering the water, the catch phase sees your hands sweep out and down, until your arms are outside the line of the shoulders and facing backward **(see figure B)**. The arms should be flexed slightly. This phase of the stroke is not propulsive, so relax your arms as much as possible to save energy.

Insweep and upsweep

The insweep is the first propulsive phase of the stroke. It begins in the catch phase and finishes under the body in the midline with your hands together (or nearly together). Keep your arms bent throughout the insweep at around 90 degrees. For the upsweep your hands circle out and back, sweeping up toward the surface, as the arms extend slightly **(see figure C)**.

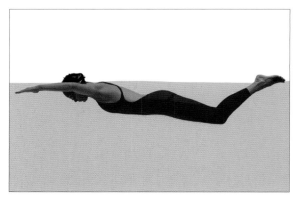

A Arms enter the water shoulder-width apart, palms facing outward.

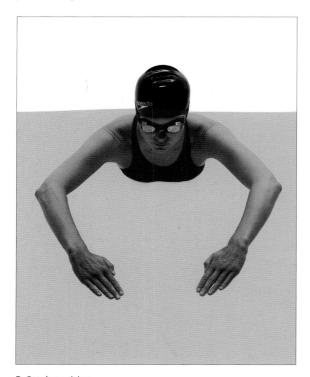

B Catch position.

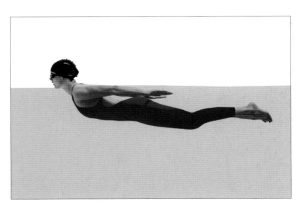

C Upsweep.

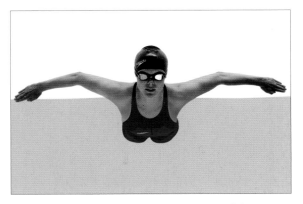

D Your arms should travel close to the surface of the water.

Release and recovery

The release begins once your hands pass your thighs (as in front crawl). At this point you should turn your palms in and extend your arms rapidly, circling them up, out and forward. Your arms should travel close to the water's surface with palms facing out until the next entry. Your arms can remain straight, although slightly bent arms are easier to achieve and more economical **(see figure D)**.

Kicking

The dolphin kick is used in the butterfly stroke. The dolphin kick is the movement of the legs in a wavelike motion, starting at the hips and moving through the legs to the feet. You should aim to keep your legs close together but not touching. One way to get the hang of the dolphin kick is to start off by kicking your legs alternately, as for front crawl, and then simply begin to move them in that same motion at the same time (you can use a float to support your upper body). A common mistake is to create a wave-like motion that is too large. Relax your kick and allow the water to dictate the position of your legs.

Coordination of the arms and legs

There are two dolphin leg kicks for every arm stroke. The first kick is larger and therefore more propulsive than the second. The two dolphin kicks should be timed as follows: kick down with the legs as the hands enter the water, and down again when they leave the water. The timing of your kicking with the arm pull is difficult, but crucial for successful butterfly swimming.

Head position and breathing

As your arms enter the water, begin to lift your head toward the surface, and continue to look up during the insweep so that your head breaks the water's surface during the upsweep. You should breathe during the upsweep and the first part of the recovery, with your face reentering the water during the second half of the recovery. A common mistake is to delay the movement of the head upward until the upsweep has finished, so be sure to start your breathing movement early. You can breathe every stroke, although competent butterfly swimmers usually breathe every two or three strokes—that is really tough!

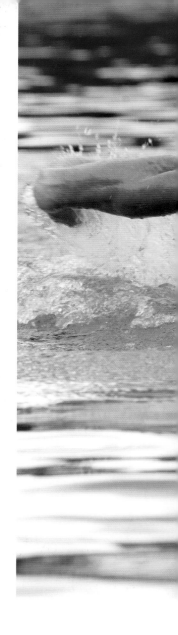

TOP TIPS FOR BUTTERFLY

- **It is all about the timing—like breast stroke, achieving a successful butterfly stroke is about the timing of your arm and leg movements.**

- **Kick twice for every arm stroke—a large kick on hand entry followed by a smaller kick at the end of the arm stroke.**

- **Keep your arms close to the water's surface during recovery.**

- **Start lifting your head early to breathe and don't lift it too high, as it wastes energy.**

- **Relax. Don't try too hard; just feel the rhythm!**

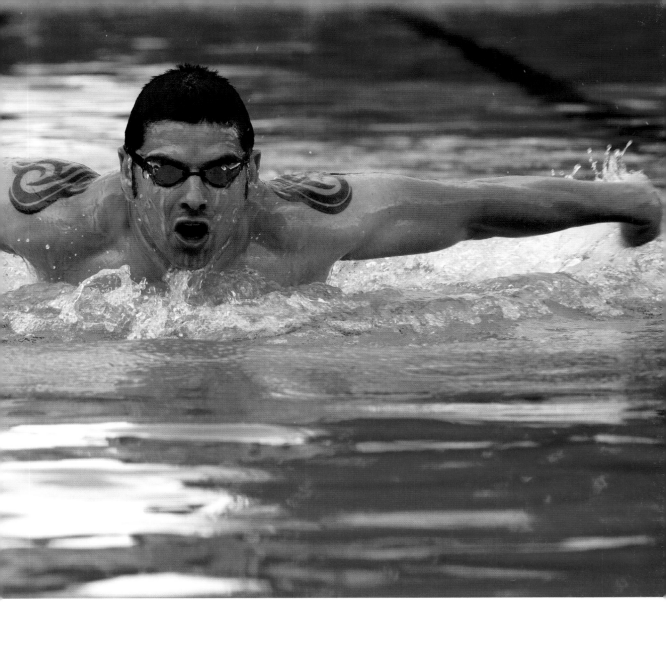

ABOVE: Tough love—butterfly is technically and physically difficult,
but once you master it you'll love showing off!

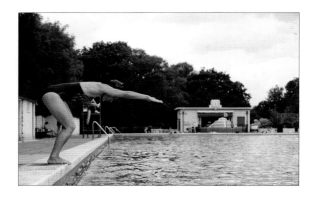 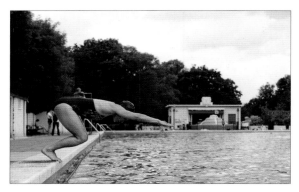

DIVING

Diving is one of those skills that a swimmer really needs—not only does it improve your times, it also looks good! The technique of diving is relatively simple in theory, but often difficult to execute in practice. Here you will find ten simple steps to help you to develop the perfect dive without those unsightly and painful belly flops!

As you become more confident, you can start with your hands by your feet or grabbing the poolside (the grab start is the fastest of the start techniques). With practice, you can start to use the full strength of your legs, making an explosive push off the wall. Or, if you are super-confident, why not try a racing start block?

10 steps to the perfect dive:

1. Make sure the pool is deep enough when you are learning to dive—I would suggest at least 8 feet depth for a beginner.

2. Curl your toes over the edge of the pool with your ankles close together (they don't need to be touching) and knees slightly bent.

3. Place your arms straight above your head, over your ears, with your thumbs clasped together.

4. Bend at the hips to ninety degrees.

5. Allow your body to fall forward and downward toward the water, about 2 – 3 feet in front of you.

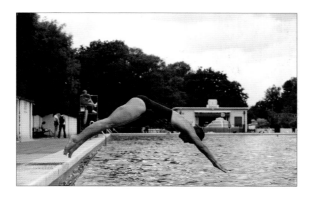

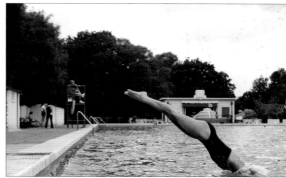

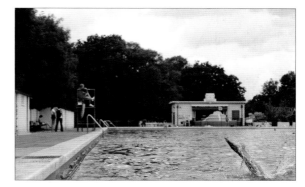

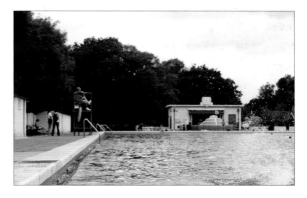

6. Just as you feel yourself falling off the edge of the poolside, straighten your legs.

7. As you enter the water, keep looking down and stretch your body out.

8. Imagine your hands are making a hole in the water and you need to get your whole body through it without making it bigger.

9. Keep your hips high and your feet higher than your hips to avoid the embarrassment of a belly flop!

10. Finally, point your hands and arms toward the surface and start to kick. Your momentum and kicking will bring you to the surface ready to start your first arm stroke.

THIS SPREAD: Diving made simple—follow the step-by-step guide and you will be impressing your friends in no time.

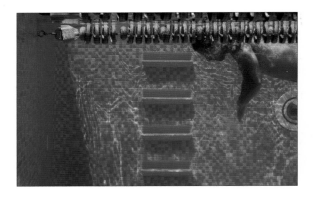 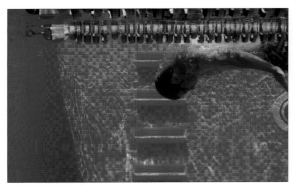

TUMBLE TURNS

One of the most poorly understood areas of swimming, the tumble turn is actually relatively easy to learn, and once mastered can significantly increase your front crawl speed. The tumble into can be divided into three phases:

- Entry
- Tumble
- Exit

Entry

As you approach the T of the line on the bottom of the pool, keep looking forward without lifting your head (focus on the line where the wall meets the bottom of the pool). Make sure you are traveling fast enough to allow yourself to tumble; if you are too slow, you will sink. You can't tumble slowly!

Tumble

With one arm outstretched, start to pull and begin to follow the hand with your head so that you curl up into a ball (like a forward roll). As you rotate, remember to breathe out of your nose so that you don't get water up your nose! Your feet should touch the wall just below the surface of the water while you remain curled up.

Exit

As soon as your feet touch the wall, extend your legs explosively. Remaining underwater, extend your body and use your hands and arms to spiral yourself back on to your front. Start kicking as soon as your feet leave the wall and, after a short glide, start your arm pull.

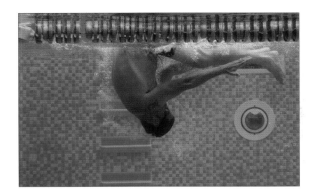

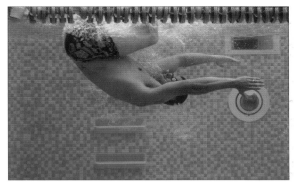

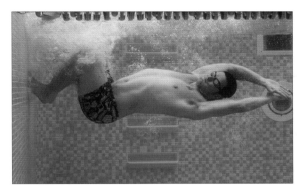

TOP TIPS FOR TUMBLE TURNS

- Start off practicing your tumble turn away from the wall if you are worried about hitting it.

- Tumble turns can be difficult to learn, but practice makes perfect! Don't give up and remember to be brave— you need to enter fast.

- As you become proficient at the tumble, aim to complete a quarter turn while doing it so that you are facing sideways (rather than up) as your feet touch the wall.

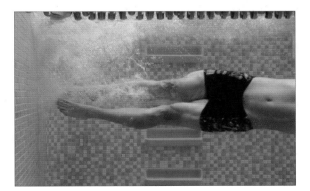

THIS SPREAD: You'll feel like a true professional when you master the tumble turn!

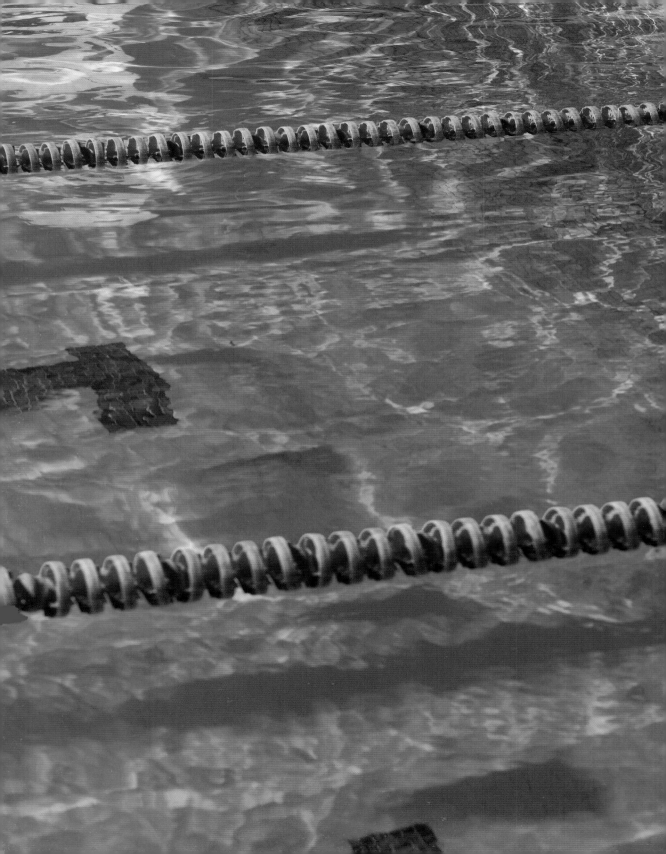

structuring
and monitoring
swimming
sessions

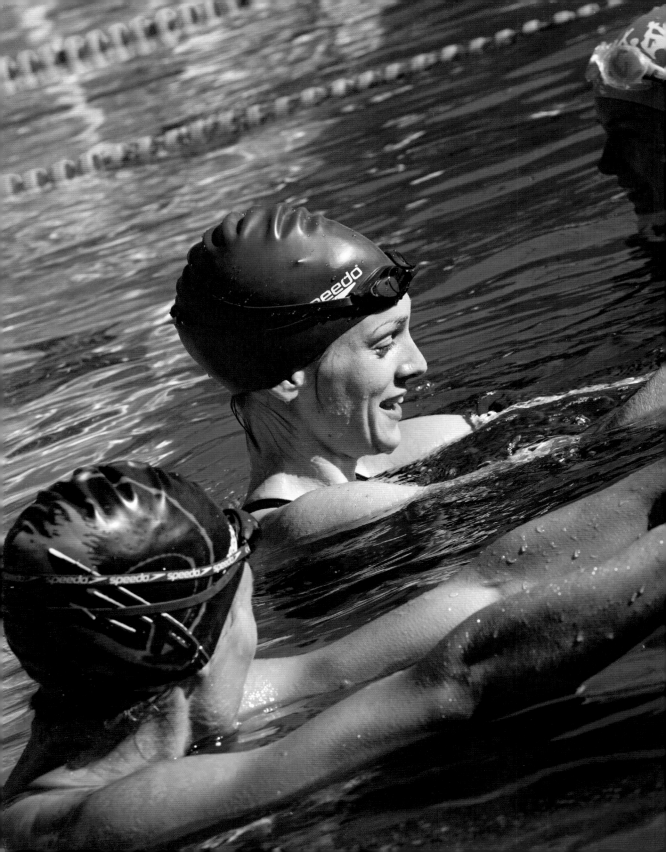

STRUCTURING SWIMS

Swimming can be incredibly tedious and boring when all you do is get into the pool and do the same old thing over and over again. Variety is the spice of life and that is as true for swimming as it is for anything else. Indeed, for many people it is often the lack of variety that leads them to drop swimming as part of their exercise routine. Let's face it, if you went to a spinning class or a step aerobics class and the instructor did the same routine to the same music every session, you would soon lose interest and stop going. So the key to success here is to plan and structure your swimming sessions to optimize both your enjoyment and performance.

The most successful exercise programs are those that are planned and well structured so that they fit in with your daily life. Identifying and committing to particular times in the week when you are going to swim will help to ensure that you don't miss sessions, and you will be more likely to maintain your swimming in the long term. Planning your swimming program with a friend so that you regularly swim together can also make a big difference—you are much less likely to miss a session that you have planned with a friend.

To maximize the benefits of swimming in the short and long term there are a number of key principles that you should keep in mind when structuring your workouts. Adhering to these will help you understand the benefits of different types of sessions and make it easy to design a program that targets those areas of fitness that are important to you.

SETTING GOALS

When designing a program think about what your goals are and what you want to achieve. Goals are personal and can vary from achieving a certain distance, to swimming a certain distance within a target time, to winning a race. Goal setting will help you to tailor your program to meet your targets, both short- and long-term, and will maximize your chance of success.

LEFT: Smile and the world smiles with you—swimming with friends is a great way to enhance your motivation and enjoyment.

By regularly monitoring and increasing how long you swim for, how hard you swim, and the number of times a week you swim (i.e. your swimming volume), you can ensure that you will progress to your goals. Setting and reaching targets will not only give you a sense of how you are progressing, it will also give you an enormous feeling of satisfaction. For more information on setting yourself goals, see page 69.

PLANNING

Planning your swimming program will optimize your performance and help to maintain the fun and excitement of swimming. In order to become fitter and improve your swimming performance, you have to work your body to a greater level than it has experienced before, forcing it to adapt, so that it is better able to cope with the stress of exercise in the future. In terms of swimming there are three key variables that you can increase in order to challenge yourself further: the number of lengths you swim, how fast you swim, and how often you swim. Together these variables make up swimming volume and give you an effective means of monitoring your swimming. (For more information, see page 56.)

You don't have to increase all of these components at once—it is much more effective to increase them one by one over time. In fact, increasing your swimming volume too quickly can result in injury because your body does not have time to adapt fully. In contrast, however, increasing your swimming volume too slowly (or not at all) often leads to boredom because you do not improve quickly enough and fail to reach your goals. This lack of success and boredom is often what leads people to stop swimming.

In Chapter 8 (page 131), I discuss training programs in more detail and you will also find a six-week program to give you an idea of how you might put a program together for yourself. You will see how I gradually increase the swimming volume by adding to the total number of lengths, the number of "hard" lengths, and the number of swims per week. Be careful when you come to increase how hard you swim, as this will increase the strain on your body the most and could lead to injury or illness if you are a bit too ambitious.

The correct speed of progression will be entirely individual—you should monitor your progression very carefully to ensure that it is happening at a rate that is right for you. Simply put, if you are continuing to improve without injury and illness, and you are enjoying your swimming, you've got it right! If you are not improving rapidly enough and are getting bored, you should make your goals more challenging; if you feel fatigued on an ongoing basis and are not enjoying swimming, make your goals a little more achievable. Make sure your plan is flexible and monitor it regularly; it should be fluid, changing to suit you as needed, not set in stone. After all, a change is as good as rest.

It is important to remember that the benefits of swimming are lost relatively quickly once you stop swimming, so make the effort to plan and structure your swimming program to keep yourself motivated. Creating goals that are both challenging and achievable, varying your program and swimming with friends are all ways in which you can maintain your swimming program throughout the year and avoid losing all the progress you have made.

RIGHT: Swimming buddies—planning your sessions with a friend will optimize your performance.

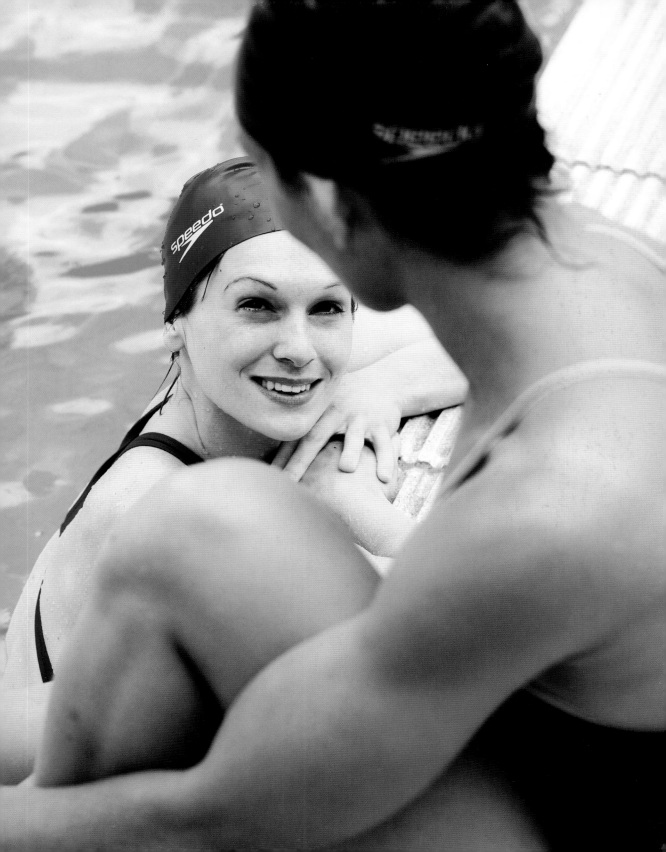

MONITORING YOUR SWIMMING

Swimming volume is measured by the total amount of swimming you complete in a set period of time (day, week, month, or year). It is made up of three components:

- how long you swim for (or how far) in a single session
- how hard (or fast) you swim
- how often you swim in a week/month

How long?

The question here is simply about how long you swim in each session. Increasing how long you swim is a great way to continue improving without having to increase how hard you are swimming, making it an easier way to increase volume. It can be measured by time or distance.

How hard?

How hard (fast) you are swimming is a measure of how much energy is demanded while swimming. Go carefully when increasing how hard you are swimming, as small increases can rapidly lead to excessive fatigue, injury and illness. On the plus side, because an increase in how hard you are swimming has such a dramatic effect on your swimming volume, you don't need to increase the number or the length of sessions as well to achieve an improvement.

SCORING A SWIMMING SESSION

How long:
1 minute = 1 point
OR
How far:
1 length = 1 point

How hard:
Easy = 1 point
Medium = 2 points
Hard = 3 points

So, fifteen minutes swimming at a hard level = 15 x 3 = 45 points.

Whereas fifteen minutes swimming at a medium level = 15 x 2 = 30 points.

And thirty lengths at an easy level = 30 x 1 = 30 points.

There are a number of different ways to gauge how hard you are swimming, some more complex and technical than others. The most common and practical ways are by observing physiological (how your body is responding, i.e. heart rate, see page 58), psychological (i.e. how you feel, see page 60) or performance (i.e. speed, see page 62) factors. There is no right or wrong method of monitoring how hard you are swimming, so choose the one that works for you.

How often?

How often you swim generally refers to the number of sessions you do in a day or a week, although longer periods of time can be used when planning long-term goals. Gradually increasing the number of times you swim in a set period is very effective in helping you to improve your swimming fitness and maintain your progress.

Calculating your swimming volume

Increasing the volume of swimming is an important factor in achieving a continuous overall improvement. Try to increase the volume of individual sessions as well as your weekly or monthly volume. Monitoring your training volume can seem very complex, but there is a simple way of allocating a point score that will give you a session-by-session volume, the accumulative total of which will give you your total swimming volume over a week, month, or year.

For a single session, rank how hard you are swimming as easy, medium, or hard and break down the time or the distance you swim for at each of these levels. Then you can use the ranking system described in the box opposite to calculate your swimming volume.

Monitoring your training volume is necessary because as you get fitter, swimming will become easier—you will find you are able to swim for longer and at an increased level of effort. In order to continue improving you must increase the difficulty so that you are challenging your body's systems. You can use this approach to monitoring your training volume to adapt and make changes to your swimming program as needed. It is also useful when it comes to setting short-term goals, i.e. achieving a certain number of points in a week.

RESPONSE TO EXERTION

The following rules may be applied as a very simple guide to your body's response to exercise:

- **EASY SWIMMING** is performed at a level that allows you to hold a full conversation during rest periods.

- **MODERATE SWIMMING** is performed at a level that allows you to hold a conversation in broken sentences and words during rest periods.

- **HARD SWIMMING** is performed at a level that only allows you to hold a conversation in single words during rest periods.

Using your heart rate to monitor how hard you are swimming

Your heart rate is a measure of how many times per minute your heart beats to pump blood around your body. During swimming you need to pump more blood around the body to provide the muscles with the oxygen and nutrients they need. Because your heart rate is closely linked to how hard you are exercising (the harder you exercise the higher your heart rate), it is a good measure of how hard you are swimming.

A person's maximum heart rate is approximately 220 minus their age. So the maximum heart rate of a forty-year-old, for example, is 220 minus 40, which equals 180 beats per minute. (Note: as we get older our maximum heart rate decreases by one beat per year on average.)

You can set levels yourself by using target heart rates. These are based on percentages of your maximum heart rate. In line with easy, medium, and hard swimming levels, heart rate targets are 60 percent, 70 percent and 80 percent of maximum heart rate respectively. So, for example, the medium (70 percent) target heart rate of a fifty-year-old man is $(220 - 50) \times 0.7 = 119$ beats per minute.

Alternatively, you can simply use the table opposite to identify your target heart rate.

Target heart rate at different intensities

Age	Easy	Medium	Hard
20	120	140	160
25	117	137	156
30	114	133	152
35	111	130	148
40	108	126	144
45	105	123	140
50	102	119	136
55	99	116	132
60	96	112	128
65	93	109	124
70	90	105	120
75	87	102	116
80	84	98	112

OPPOSITE: At the heart of the matter—feeling your carotid artery in your neck is a simple way to calculate your heart rate.

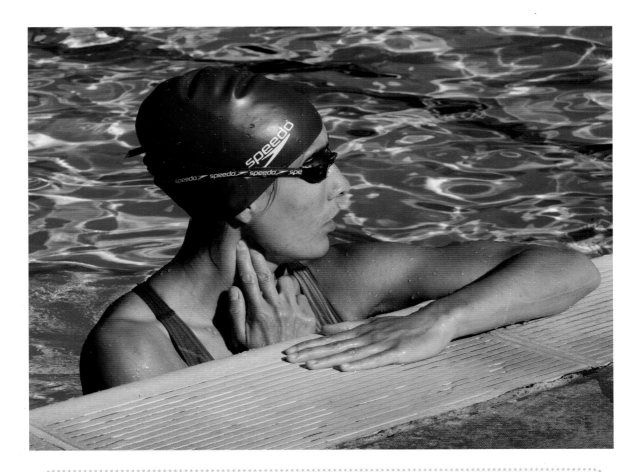

MEASURING YOUR HEART RATE

For land-based exercise the simplest way to measure heart rate is to use a heart-rate monitor. Unfortunately, however, these do not work very well when you're swimming. The water moving across the chest strap means that the signal is interrupted, and often the strap falls down. The best way to monitor your heart rate during swimming is to feel your pulse, usually at the neck or the wrist, and count the number of beats over a set period of time during rest periods using the poolside clock or a wristwatch. It is usually best to measure the number of beats over a short period of time, as your heart rate will be falling as you recover. For example, count the number of beats over six seconds, then multiply the number of beats by ten. Alternatively, you could count the number of beats over ten seconds and multiply by six.

Using the way you are feeling to monitor how hard you are swimming

By learning to grade the way you feel during exercise, you can control how hard you are swimming without the need for fancy, technical equipment. One of the simplest and most widely used techniques for doing this is through your rating of perceived exertion, or RPE. This approach relies on your ability to detect and interpret sensations from your own body; in other words, to monitor how you feel and use that information to control how hard you are working. There are a number of different scales used to rate RPE; on the right is a very simple one that you will be able to use right away. To use an RPE scale optimally, it is important to understand what the lowest and highest scores on the scale are, i.e. 1 and 10. Think about level 1 as how you feel at your most relaxed and level 10 as the feeling you have when you are swimming as fast as you can.

The more you use RPE to monitor and control how hard you are swimming, the easier it will become. For the first-time exerciser, RPE is an excellent way to make sure you are working at the right level and to learn how to listen to your body. After a while you will not even need to look at the scale to know what level you are working at.

Rating of Perceived Exertion (RPE) Scale

1   Resting (sitting down watching TV)
2
3   Very Easy
4   Easy
5
6   Medium
7
8   Hard
9
10 Maximum (the hardest you have ever exercised)

The RPE scale gives you a good indication of how hard you are swimming and how you are improving from session to session.

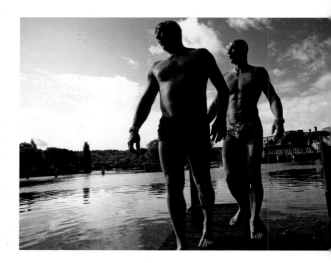

RIGHT: In at the deep end—measuring how hard you are working can be difficult in open water. This is where the RPE comes into its own.

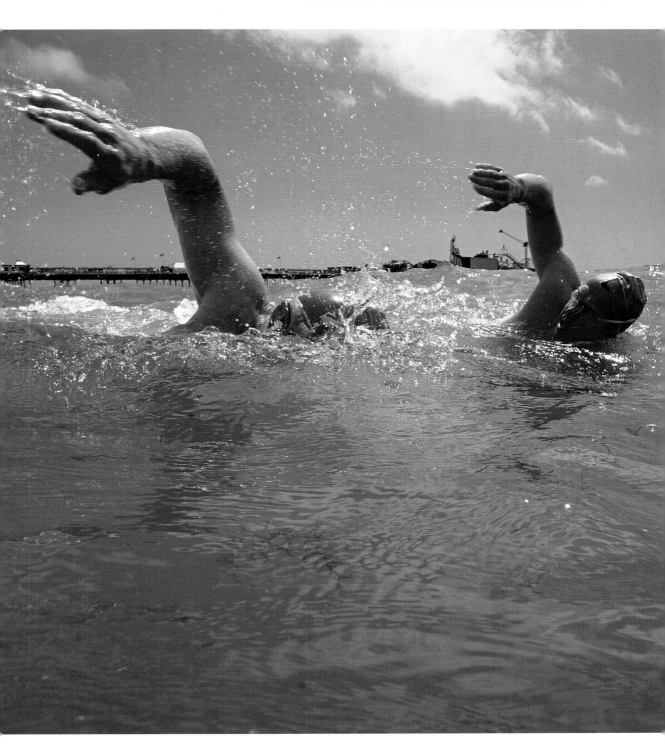

Using speed to monitor how hard you are swimming

The faster you swim, the harder you have to work, so by calculating your speed you can monitor how hard you are swimming. The easiest way to use speed as a monitor is simply to choose a set distance (number of lengths) and time yourself. Then, if you want to increase how hard you are swimming, simply speed up to reduce the period of time it takes you to complete the same number of lengths. Alternatively, you can calculate the number of lengths you swim in a set period of time and then increase the level of difficulty by increasing the number of lengths you swim during the same period of time.

To make sure that you are increasing your pace evenly across the swim, use your rating of perceived exertion (see page 60) as a guide to the amount of effort you put in during the swim. Different strokes will result in different intensities for the same speed and will vary according to your technical proficiency. Generally speaking, butterfly is by far the hardest stroke and breast stroke is usually the easiest, with front crawl and back stroke lying in the middle. You will need to set levels (speeds) for each stroke to control effectively how hard you are working during your swimming sessions.

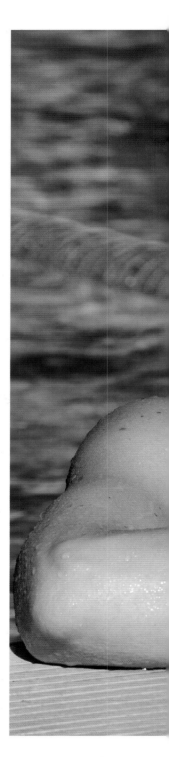

RIGHT: Having the time of your life—using a stopwatch to keep an eye on your times is a great way to monitor how hard you are working.

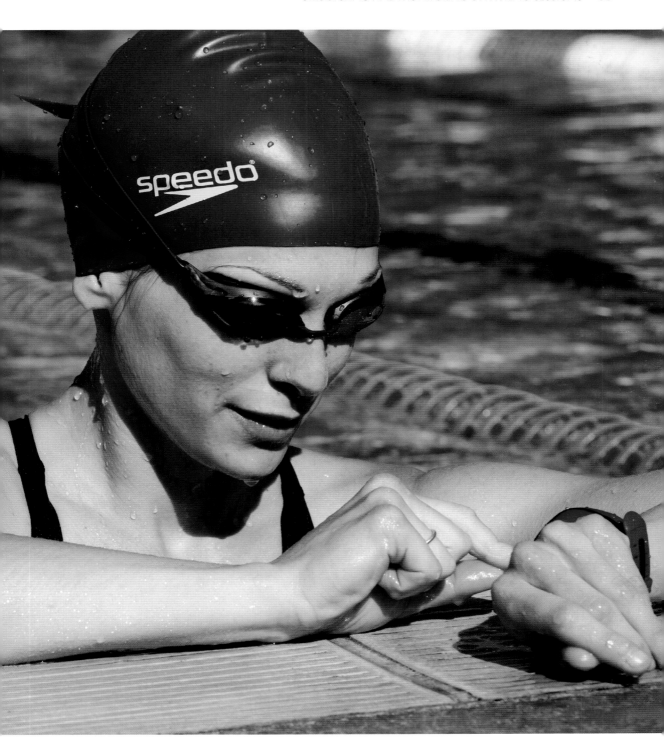

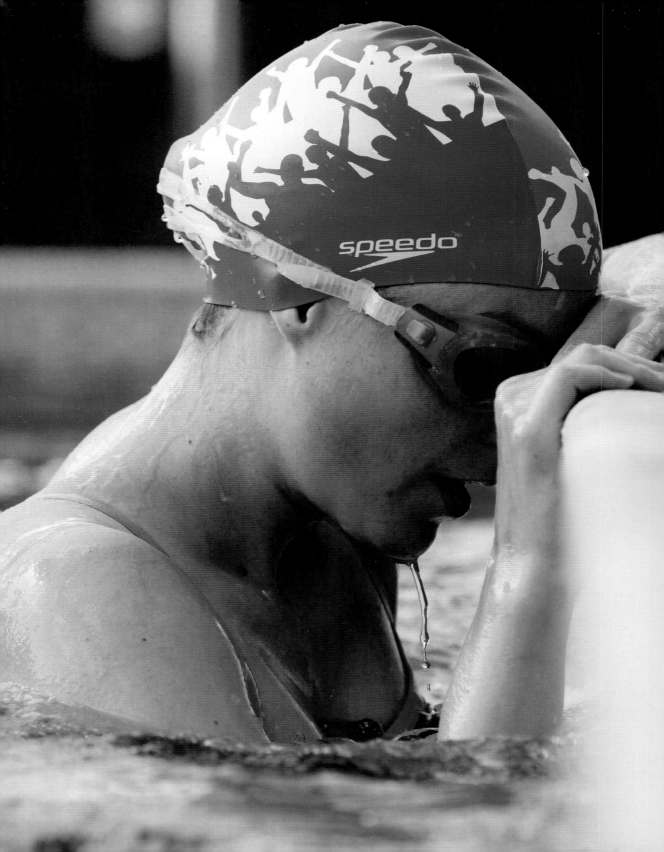

DESIGNING A PROGRAM FOR YOU

Adaptations to swimming are directly associated with the type of swimming you undertake. By designing your program in different ways you can focus on the energy systems (aerobic, speed, power), muscle groups (legs, arms, etc.) and skill/stroke (butterfly, back stroke, breast stroke, front crawl) as required. For example, swimming front crawl will improve your front crawl performance (there may also be slight progress in other strokes due to energy system changes; however, the major impact will be on your front crawl); medium-level swimming will improve your aerobic fitness, i.e. the efficiency of your lungs, heart, and muscles to use oxygen, whereas high-level swimming will improve your anaerobic capacity, i.e. your speed and strength endurance. Design your program to focus on the areas that will lead you to achieving your goal.

As well as recognizing the specificity of training, it is important to remember that we are all individuals and that our goals and responses to swimming are different. Some people will adapt very rapidly, while others adapt more slowly and require much longer periods of recovery to optimize the adaptive process. Think carefully about the volume of exercise that is appropriate for you and build in sufficient time for recovery. Seeking advice from a swimming coach/teacher or a personal trainer can be of great benefit in helping you to tailor an individual program that targets your specific needs and responses.

Rest

Giving your body time to recover is an important part of your swimming program as it will ensure that you continue to improve your fitness and avoid injury and illness. Without recovery, the body does not have time to adapt, so if you don't build enough time for this into your program you will be in a constant state of tiredness with little improvement in fitness or performance.

Listen to your body and take extra rest when you need it. A day off to recharge your batteries, both physically and mentally, is an important part of your preparation for the following week's swimming. It's a good idea to allow for some flexibility in your program, so that rather than prescribing a set day (or days) off, you play it by ear and choose when to take them based upon work or family commitments or simply how you feel. I also recommend a variable number of days between rest days, e.g. three days swimming, one day rest, four days swimming, one day rest, and so on. This instantly adds variety to your schedule, as rest days change every week and there are never more than four consecutive days of swimming.

Having said all of this, remember that too much recovery time will mean you lose the adaptations that you have gained, so strike a balance!

LEFT: Rest assured—planning recovery into your program is crucial to ensure optimal performance and avoid injury and illness.

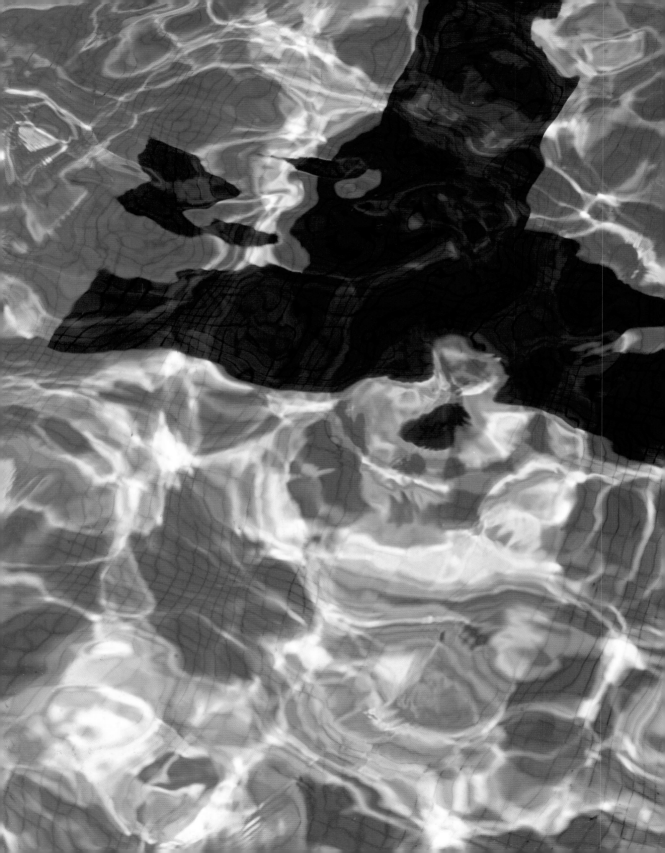

motivating
yourself

MONITOR YOUR PROGRESS

People often say to me, "Swimming is too hard; how can I make it easier?" The key is not making it easier, but simply making it more enjoyable. The fact that swimming is hard work is great; the harder it is the more calories you burn and the greater the improvement in your fitness levels. However, hard work doesn't have to be a misery, and you can adapt your exercise program to ensure that it is challenging but enjoyable. Plus, swimming is a great exercise for setting goals because as you improve your technique you can achieve new distances or achieve faster times for set distances.

The reason swimming is hard work is because it is highly technical and you are using the relatively small muscles of the arms (unlike in running or cycling). Even with an improved stroke it can still be hard work, but you will find you can swim at the same speed with more ease. With an improved technique, you can swim faster and farther for the same effort. Nothing good comes easy—but you can still enjoy it!

"Swimming is boring!"

How often do I hear this? And there is no doubt about it, swimming can be boring if you do the same thing every time you get into the water (swimmers often refer to the boredom of staring at the bottom of the pool as "Black Line Disease"). There are, however, a variety of different ways in which you can eliminate boredom and enjoy swimming every time you go.

RIGHT: Black line disease—adding variety into your session is a surefire way to avoid boredom.

Set yourself goals

Having a target to aim for is one of the best ways to eliminate boredom and motivate yourself. Clearly identifying a goal that you want to achieve, whether it's to lose weight, to swim a mile, to reduce lower-back pain, or just to look great, will be invaluable in making swimming more fun and enjoyable.

When setting goals, you should have both short-term targets (i.e. goals to be achieved within a week or a month) and long-term ones (those that you hope to achieve within six months to a year). A sensible short-term goal, for example, would be to swim a certain distance in a set period of time. The more physical targets, such as weight loss or increased strength, should form part of your longer-term strategy, as they may take a little longer to achieve—say three to six months. Setting physical-outcome goals over shorter periods than this is more likely to be unsuccessful because of the time it takes for your body to change, and it will probably lead to a loss of motivation if you feel like progress isn't quick enough.

So make sure that all your goals are achievable yet challenging. If they are too easy you will get bored and if they are too difficult you will lose interest; either way you will probably give up on your swimming program.

Reward yourself

Reward yourself when you reach your goals (both short- and long-term). Make sure the reward is something that you really want, but do not allow yourself to have it if you have not reached your goal. The reward should reflect the achievement and should recognize the effort required to reach the goal. So short-term goals should earn smaller rewards, say an extra hour in bed, while a long-term goal might be rewarded with something more substantial, such as a new gadget or item of clothing (avoid rewarding yourself with food, though).

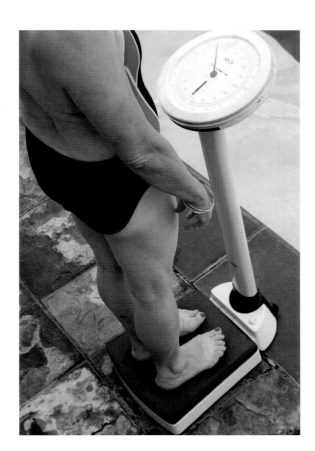

ABOVE: Make sure your goals are realistic and achievable to avoid setting yourself up for failure.

Swim with others

Swimming on your own can sometimes be a lonely experience. A great way to enhance your enjoyment is to swim with others, because although you do spend much of the time with your head submerged in the water, there are still lots of opportunities to chat.

Having a swimming buddy, someone you regularly swim with, can increase your enjoyment of exercise and help you maintain your swimming program. On days when you don't feel like swimming your swimming buddy will encourage you, and vice versa, meaning that you are much more likely to achieve your short- and long-term-goals. Sharing goals with your swimming buddy is also a great way to enhance motivation and improve your chances of success. It can be helpful to arrange to meet at the same time and place each week, so that you will have to attend the session to avoid letting your friend down.

Join a swimming club

You are never too old to join a swimming club, and there are over 450 Masters Swimming clubs in the United States, with over 50,000 members. Masters Swimming is swimming for adults that encompasses the whole range of ability from casual fitness swimming to highly organized competitive swimming. To qualify as a "Masters" swimmer the only requirement is that you are over eighteen years of age (there is no upper age limit). Since its establishment in the United States in the late 1970s, Masters Swimming has become a major sport globally. Masters Swimming competitions are divided into age categories starting with 18–24 years and moving upward. Unlike competitive age-group swimming, Masters Swimming events rarely require qualifying times, so if you want to compete you can simply join a club, send in your entry, and away you go!

That said, there are many other reasons to join a swimming club besides competing. In fact, the majority of Masters swimmers rarely compete. Swimming classes, camaraderie, and lots of fun are some of the other reasons why joining a swimming club might be a great way for you to enhance your enjoyment of swimming.

RIGHT: Swimming buddies—take the opportunity to swim with others and make swimming a sociable event as well as a workout.

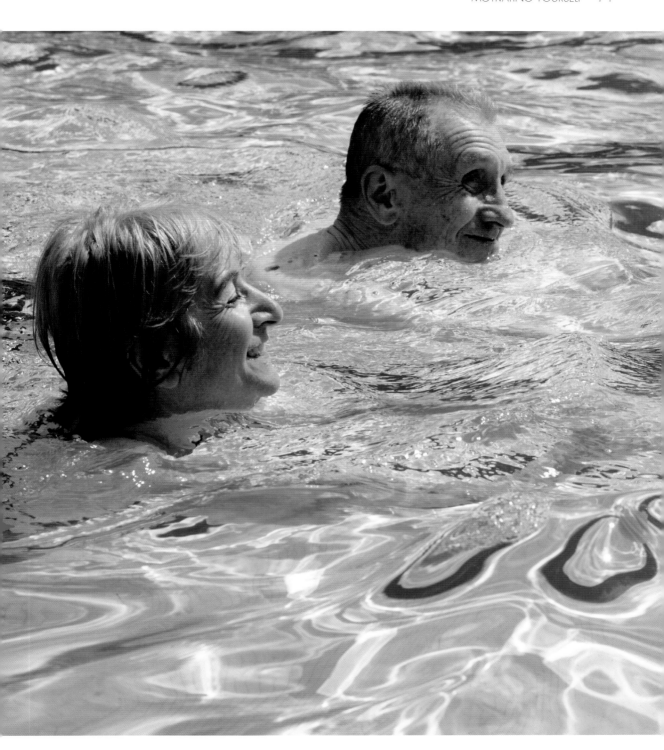

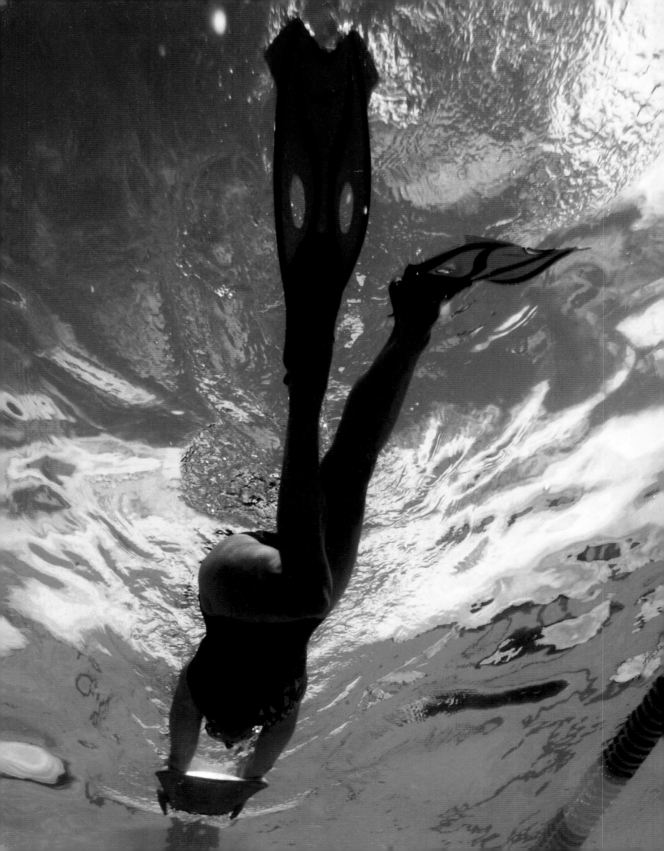

Pick and mix your strokes

Swimming the same stroke for the same number of lengths every time you get in the water is the quickest route to boredom! To increase interest, use all of the strokes. Don't be afraid of trying a new stroke for the first time—you may find it difficult at first but you will soon get the hang of it. Learning to swim a new stroke is highly motivating and, having learned it, setting goals to achieve faster speeds and longer distances can help sustain your drive.

Designing your swimming program so that every session is different will keep you enthused. You can also concentrate on different parts of a stroke—arms only (often termed "pulling") or legs only (often termed "kicking")—which will add variety and make you work harder.

Use different speeds

You can easily add interest to your swimming session by varying your speed. Try the following methods to vary the level of your sessions:

Negative split

Divide your session into two halves and make the second half harder than the first. Alternatively, divide the workout into as many blocks as you wish and make each period of time or length harder than the previous one. For example, divide your fifty-length swim into five ten-length blocks and try to swim each ten lengths faster than the previous ten. Or you could divide a thirty-minute swim into three lots of ten minutes and try to swim more lengths with each ten minutes.

Speed play (fartlek)

Speed play (or "fartlek" in Swedish) is a form of continuous exercise that incorporates short periods of medium or hard effort interspersed with periods of easy swimming. So you might repeat a cycle of five lengths of hard swimming, followed by five lengths of easy swimming for thirty minutes. Or you could try five minutes at a medium level, five minutes easy, ten minutes medium, and finish with ten minutes easy. You can choose any combination of time and/or lengths to make up your session.

Intervals

Divide your workout into periods of swimming, usually medium or hard levels, interspersed with periods of rest. For example, ten five-length blocks at a medium level with one-minute rests between each. Alternatively, try swimming twenty single lengths at a hard level with a thirty-second recovery between each.

LEFT: On the flipside—using flippers adds variety and improves the strength of your legs and feet.

GADGETS AND GIZMOS

There are a number of swimming aids that can add variety to your program:

- Hold a float to concentrate your efforts on kicking—work on your flutter kick, dolphin kick, or breast stroke kick (this can be very hard work, which is a good thing!)
- Wear flippers while kicking only or during normal swimming to increase the work of your legs (it is important to select the right length of flipper—the longer the flipper, the more stress you place on your ankles).
- Place a pull-buoy between your legs to concentrate effort on your arms only (often termed "pulling").
- Use hand paddles or aquatic mitts to increase the surface area of your hand and make it more difficult to pull—great for strength and strength endurance.
- Use finger paddles to strengthen your hands and forearms.
- If you really want to work those arms, try a drag suit (a very large, baggy costume) or wearing a T-shirt for extra drag.
- A really tough technique is to tie your ankles together or drag a bucket tethered around your waist—however, this is only for the advanced.

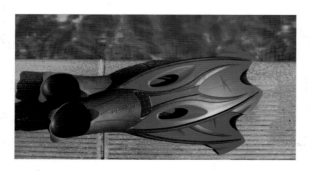

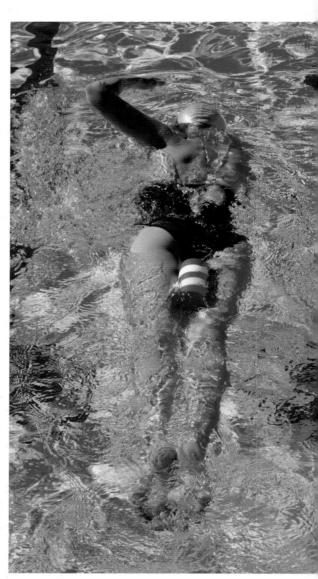

THIS SPREAD: Variety is the spice of swimming—using pull-buoys, paddles, and flippers can add variety and also improve your performance.

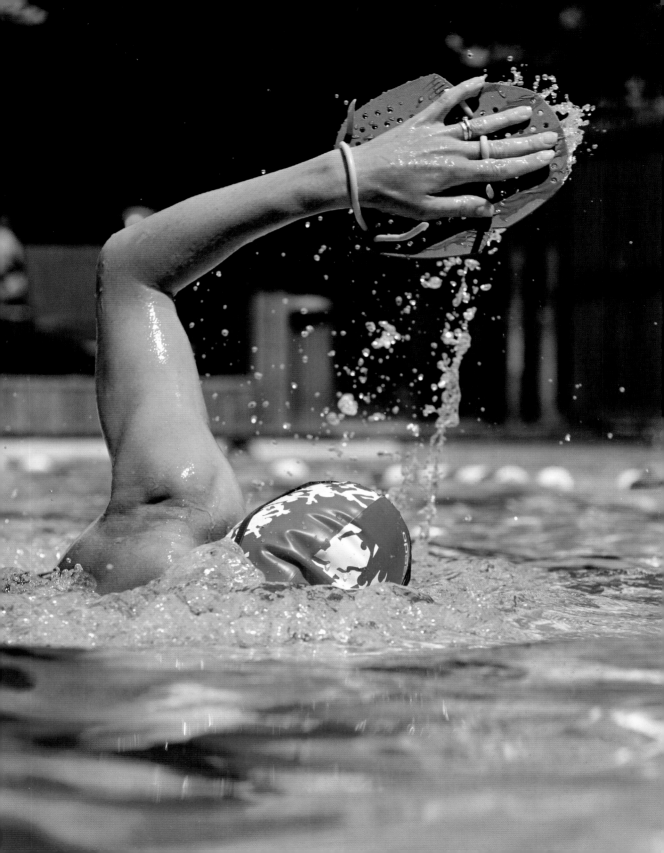

Exercise with music

Research has shown that listening to music can improve the quality of your workout, increase your overall enjoyment, and help to maintain your exercise program in the long term. And, believe it or not, you can now buy waterproof MP3 players to use when swimming.

Music is particularly useful for sustained low- or medium-level swimming when it can make the exercise feel easier and, in so doing, increase your enjoyment. Why not make your own compilation for your MP3, selecting tracks that have a motivating effect for you. Use as many tracks as you can and listen to them on "shuffle" mode to keep things interesting. If you don't have a waterproof MP3 player, why not listen to some stirring music before you swim to get motivated and energized for your session!

TOP MOTIVATING TUNES

"Fire Starter"—Prodigy
"Lose Yourself"—Eminem
"Baby Fratelli"—The Fratellis
"Dreamland"—Robert Miles
"What's Up"—4 Non Blondes
"Carmina Burana"—Orff
"Lacrimosa (Requiem in D Minor)"—Mozart

BELOW: Underwater MP3 players now allow you to swim to the beat of your favorite music. RIGHT: Kick the habit—by focusing on kicking and pulling you can add variety and improve performance all at the same time.

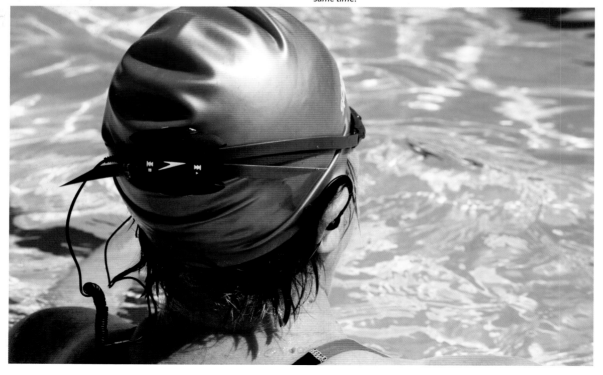

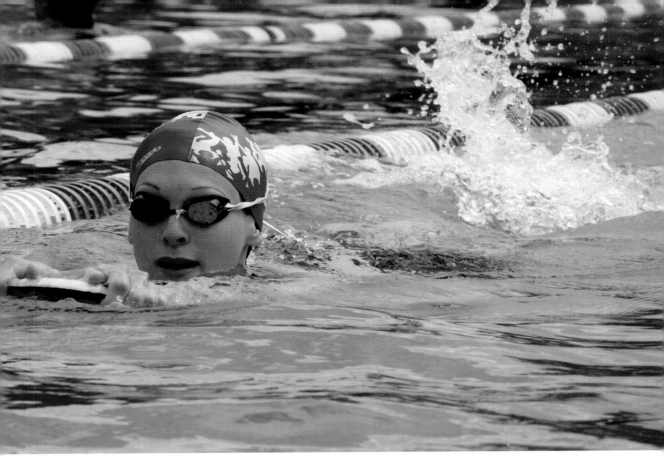

MONITOR YOUR PROGRESS

Keeping track of your progress is a great way to motivate yourself. The easiest way to monitor your performance is by using time trials (racing against the clock). You can choose any distance you feel comfortable with for time trials; however, using longer distances, such as 400 meters, 800 meters or 1500 meters make it easier to note any changes in performance because you are swimming for a longer period of time. Alternatively, you can choose to swim for a set period of time and see how far you can swim, e.g. how many lengths you can cover in twenty minutes (often termed a T20) or thirty minutes (a T30).

In addition to time trials, you can use the development of new strokes as a way to monitor your progress. When you first start swimming you usually choose your favored stroke and stick to it. By mastering a stroke and then moving on to learning and mastering another you can keep tabs on your technical progress, and you can then use time trials for the different strokes to monitor your physical progress.

Another way to watch your progress as you become a proficient swimmer is to join a swimming club and enter races.

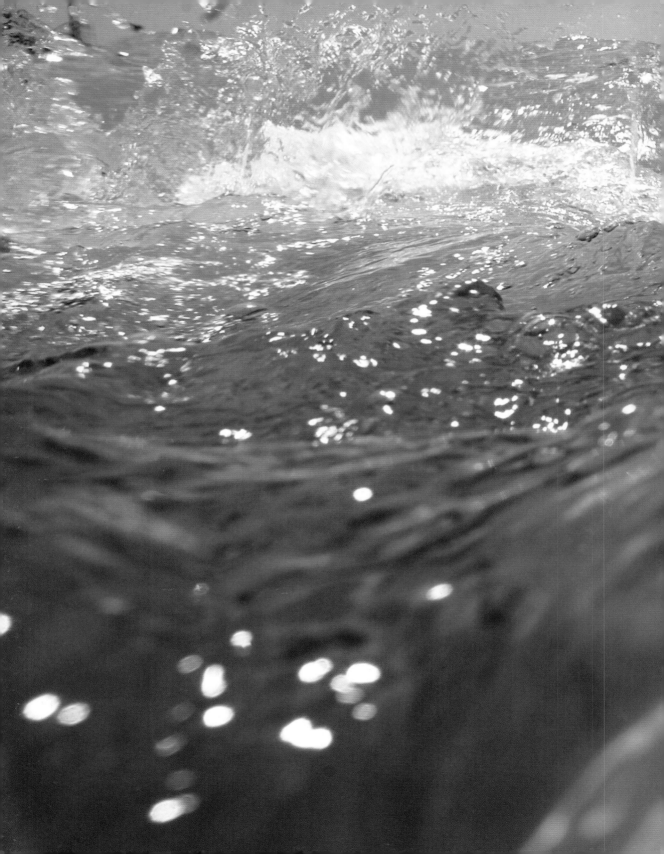

open-water

swimming

GET OUT IN THE OPEN

Swimming in open waters (rivers, lakes and seas) is one of the most liberating, spectacular and exciting experiences. However, it can also be a scary, intimidating environment if you are not geared up for it, and preparation is critical for a safe and enjoyable open-water swim. So who can do it? How, when, where and why? Read on to find out.

Who?

Swimmers of most standards can take to the open water, although you do need to be reasonably proficient and comfortable in the water in order to be safe, particularly when swimming in the sea. It is also of the utmost importance that you always swim open water with others, never alone.

How?

Most open-water swimming is performed using the front crawl or breast stroke with a few technical changes compared to pool swimming. Being able to navigate and having the ability to lift your head to sight where you are going is fundamental to open-water swimming. In addition, it's important to get used to swimming in a wetsuit to optimize performance, as this also requires a subtly different technique.

When?

You can swim open water at any time of the year. Even on the coldest winter day you will find open-water swimmers dipping into lakes, rivers and seas around the country. Of course you do need to be wary of the cold, but by reducing the time you spend in the water or wearing a wetsuit (and sometimes neoprene gloves, boots, and a hat in very cold water) you can safely swim all year round.

Why?

You can swim for pleasure or you can race in one of a large number of open water swimming races around the country (see Resources, page 140). At the 2008 Olympic Games in Beijing open water swimming had its debut, marking the growth in popularity of open water swimming.

Where?

You can swim just about anywhere there is open water, but great care must be taken as there may be unseen dangers, including strong currents, dense weeds/seaweed, submerged objects, etc. The best way to swim safely in open water is to swim at designated open-water swimming sites/centers and with an open water swimming club. There are hundreds of dedicated sections of lakes, rivers and sea for open water swimming and as many clubs. There are also a number of open water swimming associations that organize swims across iconic bodies of water including the English Channel, the Solent, the Gibraltar Straits from Europe to Africa, and the Hellespont from Europe to Asia (see Resources, page 140).

RIGHT: To wetsuit or not to wetsuit—it's your choice. Wetsuits are a great way to keep warm, but you might prefer to go au naturel.

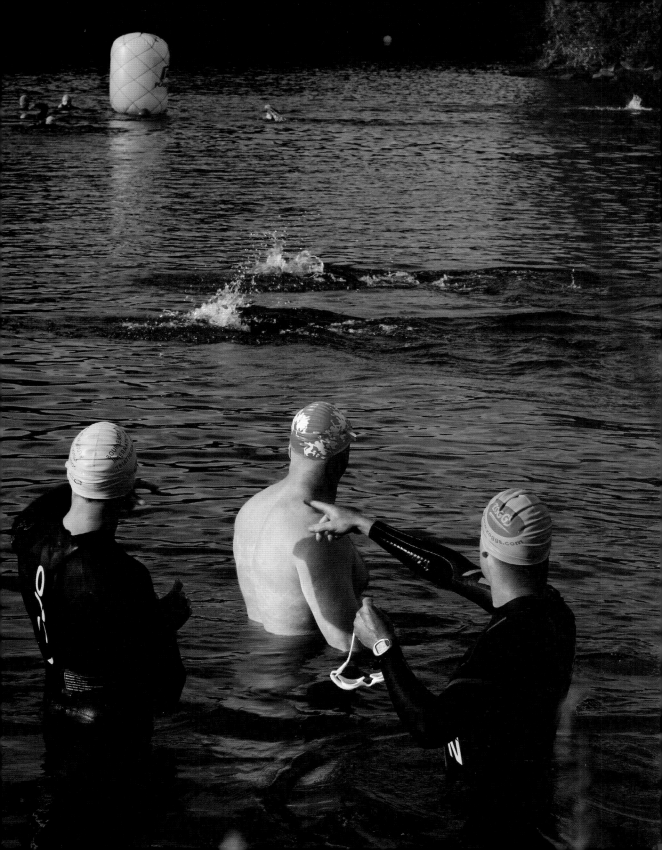

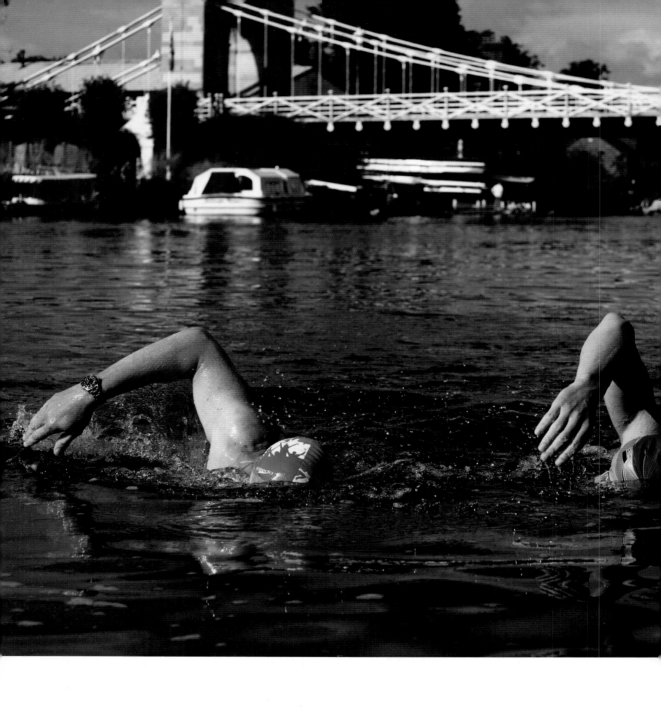

*ABOVE: Two's company—never swim alone in open water, even
when you are close to shore.*

Swimming adventure vacations

A great way to breathe new life into your swimming, improve your techniques and—most importantly—have lots of fun is to take a swimming adventure vacation. There are a small number of companies that offer swimming vacations in some of the most idyllic destinations in the world, including the Mediterranean, the Caribbean, the Middle East and Northern Europe (see Resources, page 140). You don't have to be a highly accomplished swimmer to go on this type of holiday; most cater to all standards and you will always find someone of a similar level on the trip. When I was preparing David Walliams and the *This Morning* girls for the English Channel, we went away to Croatia, Malta (Gozo) and the British Virgin Islands for training. These were amazing trips, and we swam in warm waters, surrounded by the exotic flora and fauna of the sea. There is no better way to bring back the enjoyment of swimming than to do it in the open water in new and exotic locations.

OPEN-WATER SWIMMING TECHNIQUE

The most common strokes used for open water swimming are the front crawl and breast stroke (it is unlikely that you will swim back stroke and butterfly in open water). The basics of the swimming strokes do not change in open water. However, the one big technical change with open-water swimming is sighting (seeing where you are going). Unlike in a pool, where there are black lines and lane ropes to guide you, swimming in a straight line can be very difficult in open water. You will need to lift your head while swimming to see where you are going. A great tip is to pick a point on the bank (if you're in a river or lake) or a boat or pier (if you're in the sea), and use that marker as your target. Try to only lift your head every ten strokes or so, as it can be very tiring (you can increase this as you become more proficient).

If you are wearing a wetsuit your technique may also have to change a little, as your arm and shoulder movements may be restricted, even in individually tailored suits. You may find this tiring at first, but it soon passes with practice.

In general, swimming in open water can be more strenuous because you do not get the opportunity to rest at the end of each length—there aren't any!—and you have to keep looking where you are going. The important thing is to relax and try to save as much energy as possible. Once you've overcome these initial obstacles you will find being in the open water an exhilarating way to swim.

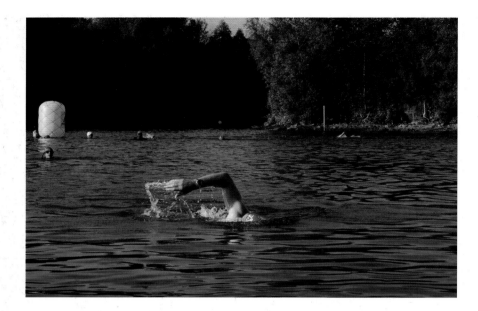

THIS SPREAD: Distances can be deceptive in open water— make sure you plan your swims carefully and never go out alone.

MONITORING YOUR SWIMMING

· ·

We've already looked at measuring your swimming volume when you are in the pool by monitoring how long, how hard and how often you are swimming (see pages 56–57). However, monitoring your swimming volume is much more complex in open water because it can be a lot more difficult to assess how far and how hard you are swimming.

In open water it is therefore crucial that you learn to use the rating of perceived exertion (RPE) method (see page 60). This will allow you to monitor how hard you are swimming on a constant basis.

It is usually possible to estimate how far you are swimming in rivers and lakes but is much more difficult in the sea. In these cases, rather than measuring the distance you are swimming, you need to measure how long you are swimming for.

Keeping track of your progress in open water swimming is also a bit more of a challenge. The best way to do it is to select a number of set distance swims and regularly time yourself over each of these.

Although it takes a bit of organization and forward planning, being able to measure your swimming volume and how you are progressing is as important in open water as it is in the swimming pool—it will help you to avoid injury and illness and keep you motivated.

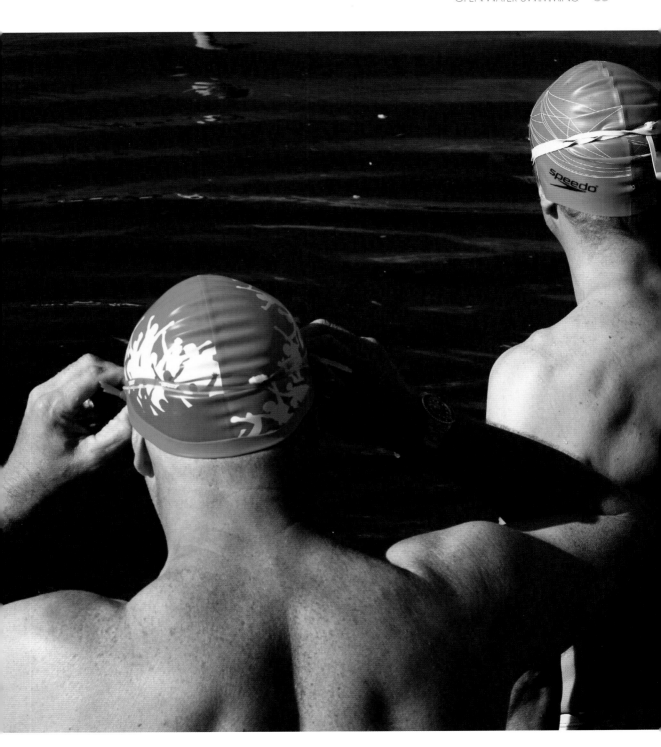

TAKING PRECAUTIONS

Will I need a wetsuit?

Wetsuits simply add an additional layer of insulation, helping to reduce the loss of body heat to the cold water. While the open-water swimming community tends to frown upon the use of wetsuits, they can be a very sensible addition to your swimming equipment, especially if you are likely to be seriously affected by the cold. They will also make you more buoyant.

Making sure your wetsuit fits correctly is essential. An ill-fitting wetsuit can lead to poor insulation and significant abrasions, sores, and open wounds. Having a wetsuit made to measure is the best way to ensure comfort and optimal performance; there are a number of swimming equipment manufacturers who provide such a service (see Resources, page 140).

Use a lubricant

Abrasions caused by the prolonged rubbing of a wetsuit on skin, or by skin on skin, can make open water swimming a misery. Make sure you use some form of lubricant like petroleum jelly in the areas most likely to be affected by rubs and sores (i.e. the neck, under the arms, and between the legs). This will make your experience much more enjoyable!

Use ear plugs

Cold, unchlorinated open water can cause ear infections (chlorine kills the bacteria that commonly cause ear infections). Wearing earplugs and using over-the-counter ear drops can help you avoid problems.

Tinted goggles

Choosing the right goggles is very important in open water. They need to be as comfortable as possible (a snug fit without being too tight) because you will be wearing them nonstop for long periods of time. You will also need to pick the appropriate tint on the lenses. On dull, overcast days you will need clear goggles to improve vision. In contrast, on bright sunny days you will need a dark tint or reflective lenses to reduce glare and avoid sore eyes. I always recommend having a number of pairs of goggles with varying tints in your kit bag so that you are ready for anything!

Avoid sunburn

During open water swimming you may experience significant exposure to the sun, so make sure you use a high SPF, waterproof sunscreen. You should always wear sunscreen in open-air pools and the beach, too.

Hydration

The combination of cold water, high salinity, and sun can lead to rapid dehydration and glycogen depletion in open water. Unlike when you're in the swimming pool, you don't have the opportunity to stop after each length and take in some fluid. You will need to think very carefully about how you will feed yourself in open water (using a circular route to the bank/jetty/shore or having a boat alongside). Furthermore, deciding what you eat and drink is not always a simple task, as saltwater can often make your favorite food or drink taste terrible!

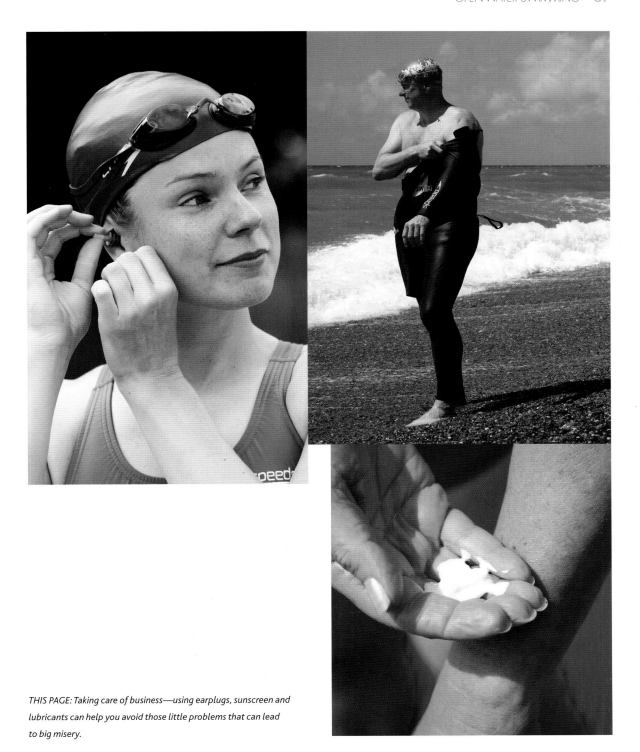

THIS PAGE: Taking care of business—using earplugs, sunscreen and lubricants can help you avoid those little problems that can lead to big misery.

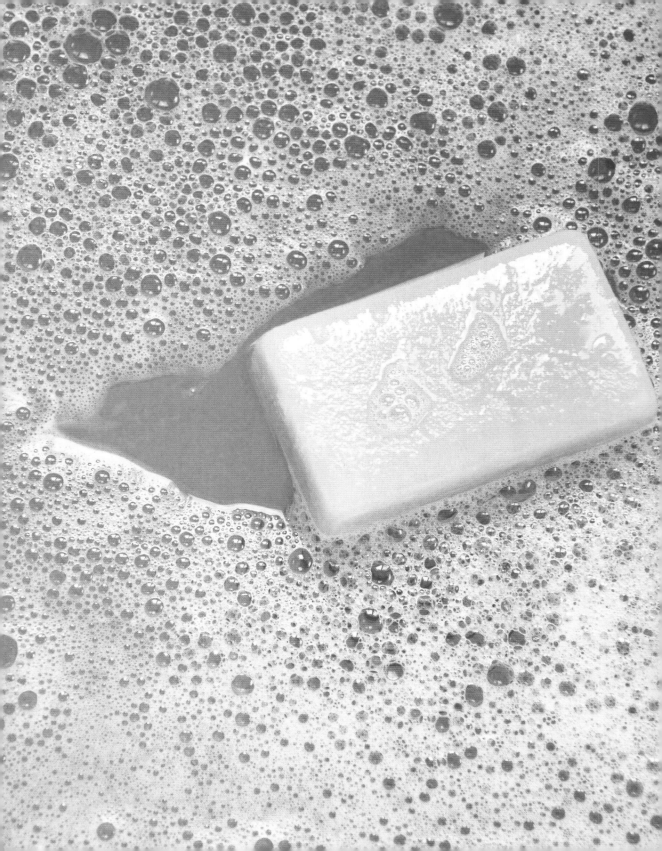

looking after
yourself

TAKING CARE OF YOURSELF

Swimming is a great form of exercise because it uses all of your muscles and gives you whole-body toning. That said, it is worth taking some time to look after yourself when you are not in the water too. Land training exercises will help your body cope with the demands of swimming, and ensuring you take good care of your skin, hair, and diet will mean that you look great as well as feel great.

Swimsuit care

Chlorine (or rather the hypochlorite ion that is formed from chlorine in water) causes fabrics to fade quickly when not rinsed off immediately after swimming. It can also affect the elasticity of your suits, resulting in a sad, faded, saggy suit—not your most attractive look! Rinse your suits in fresh water and dry after every swim in order to avoid having to continually replace them.

Skin care

Swimming can really take its toll on your skin because of the chemicals (mainly chlorine) used to keep pools free of bacteria. Chlorine strips moisture and oils from your skin; it is therefore not unusual for it to become dry, itchy and irritated. In fact, this form of chemical dermatitis is such a common problem that it's been dubbed "swimmer's itch" (see box opposite for how to prevent it). Saltwater has a similar effect on the skin, particularly on hot, sunny days.

Occasionally a rash may develop that is more problematic, producing blisters resembling chicken pox. Such rashes are normally caused by bacteria that are particularly prevalent in hot tubs and jacuzzis. These rashes will usually disappear without treatment after seven to ten days, unless complications such as infections develop. Any such infections of the skin or other parts of the body need to be examined and treated by a doctor. Skin rashes may also develop when swimming in open water due to parasites in the water. Don't panic, though, serious skin problems are rare!

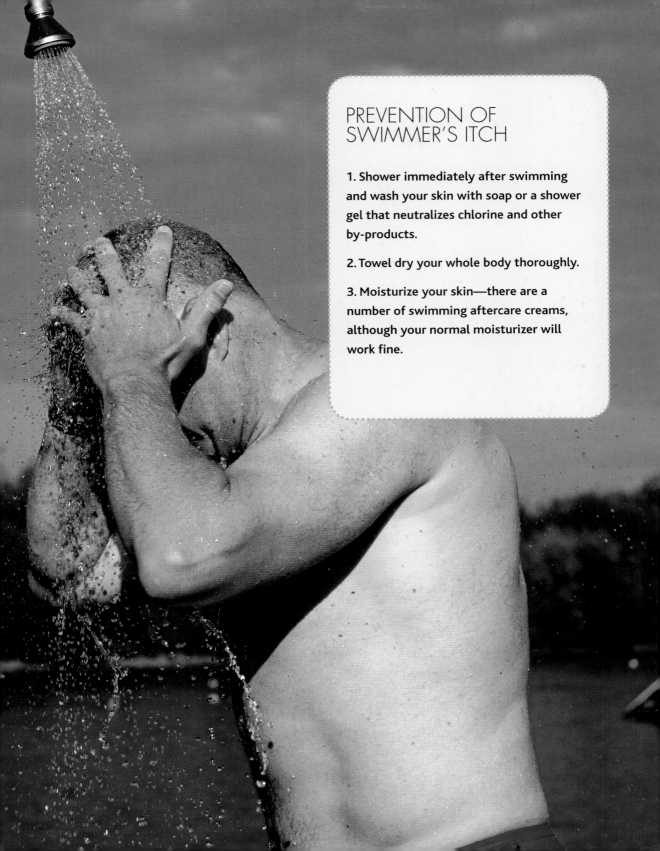

PREVENTION OF SWIMMER'S ITCH

1. Shower immediately after swimming and wash your skin with soap or a shower gel that neutralizes chlorine and other by-products.

2. Towel dry your whole body thoroughly.

3. Moisturize your skin—there are a number of swimming aftercare creams, although your normal moisturizer will work fine.

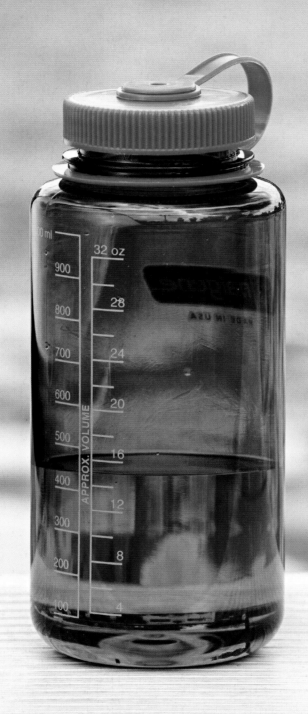

Hair care

Chlorine in swimming pools strips moisture from your hair and can leave it dry, brittle, and smelling of chlorine. There are a range of special swimming shampoos on the market which remove chlorine and its odor from the hair. Many of them will also help to remove copper deposits and other oxidized metals present in swimming pool water that can cause lighter colored hair to take on a greenish tint. The myth that blond (bleached) hair goes green after swimming is in fact true—I like to call it "chlorine green"! It is easily returned to its normal color in the shower with special shampoo though. In addition to removing chlorine and oxidized metals, swimming shampoos also clean and condition the hair in the same way as normal shampoos, but additional conditioning may be necessary for very dry, brittle hair. Another alternative is to wear a swimming cap to reduce your hair's exposure to the water; this will also save you time washing and drying your hair on busy days.

Preventing injury

It is essential to look after your muscles and joints. If you haven't swum before, are returning to swimming after a long time out of the water, or are swimming a large number of sessions, you may pick up minor discomforts that can lead to more problematic injuries. Common problem areas are the shoulders, back, and neck. Don't ignore soreness and pain that is localized in a certain muscle or joint—act early and you can often avoid injury. Take a couple of days off swimming, replacing sessions with land work and flexibility before returning to the pool for some light swimming. If the problem gets worse or continues for a long time, seek help from a qualified massage therapist or physical therapist.

Prevention is the best cure, so stick to your program of strength and flexibility (see pages 97–129) and don't forget to have a light stretch before and after every swim.

Land training

The concept of cross-training—using a variety of training methods to enhance your performance—is very beneficial to swimmers. Land training is commonly used by competitive swimmers because it improves strength, strength endurance, and flexibility, as well as reducing the risk of injury and combating boredom. All of these reasons apply to the recreational swimmer too. Don't be afraid to venture into the gym or join a circuit-training class; it could enhance your performance and will certainly add variety to your workouts. (See Chapter 7 for a variety of land training exercises.)

Hydration

It always seems a little bizarre to be concerned about hydration when you are submerged in water. However, dehydration is very common in swimmers for a number of reasons. Swimming requires a lot of energy and in keeping up with your body's energy demands you produce a large amount of heat that you have to lose in order to keep your body temperature within a safe range. The best way to lose this heat is by sweating—yes, believe it or not, you sweat when you are swimming! However, because you are in a wet environment you are not aware of how much you are sweating and so it is easy to become dehydrated. That is why it is important to ensure you are fully hydrated before you get in the water and that you have a drink when you get out of the water to help rehydrate (alcohol is not very effective for rehydration; a water based drink is required!). If you are going to be in the water for a long time you should take a bottle to the poolside and drink during your session.

OPPOSITE: Water, water everywhere—despite being submerged in water you can dehydrate rapidly when swimming, so make sure you have a drink handy.

Diet

In general, your muscles require carbohydrates as fuel for exercise. That's why it is important to make sure you have a full store of carbohydrates in your muscles (called muscle glycogen) and other parts of your body. If you are swimming regularly at a high level for prolonged periods you should consider consuming carbohydrates before, during, and after your swim.

Before swimming

Large meals should be eaten at least 1–2 hours before a training session, but you can eat small amounts of energy-rich carbohydrate foods, such as chocolate, fruit, cookies, or energy bars at any point before a swim. These foods all have a high glycemic index (GI), which means that the glucose appears in your blood very quickly, making them great snacks for exercise. Eating snacks during the thirty-minute period before you get in the water will optimize their value as a fuel source for your swimming session. By eating a small amount of high-GI food you can ensure optimal energy without causing cramps or feeling sick.

During swimming

If you are swimming for long durations you will need some form of sustenance. Unfortunately, it can be difficult to eat while swimming—not only is there little time to chew, but mixing food with chlorinated water or saltwater makes it taste terrible! The best source of carbohydrates during swimming will be in the form of energy drinks, which allow you to maintain your carbohydrate levels and rehydrate at the same time. There are lots of commercially available energy drinks on the market, which generally contain between 4 and 12 percent carbohydrate, which is perfect for exercise. They are easy to consume, but it is important to choose a product and a flavor that you like when you are swimming (and remember—mixed with chlorinated water or saltwater, it can taste very different). You can also make your own drinks by mixing fruit juices with water but beware of fruit juices—they can upset your tummy.

After swimming

Try to consume carbohydrates within thirty minutes of finishing a swimming session—this period after exercise is the most effective time for your body to store carbohydrates (if you can't eat immediately after swimming, keep your energy drink going). Replenishing your carbohydrate store after swimming is an investment in your next session: if you don't fully replete your energy stores after exercise your next swim will suffer.

Weight loss

I know what you are thinking— "carbohydrates are calories!" And you are right. If weight loss is your aim, reduce the amount of carbohydrates you consume, but don't cut them out completely. Carbohydrates are vital in maintaining the quality of each swimming session, and they are unlikely to be stored as fat when consumed alongside exercise. And remember, even if you are trying to lose weight, optimal hydration is crucial for health and performance—so make sure you drink when you exercise.

RIGHT: Food for thought—planning your diet can help you stay healthy and energized for swimming and for life.

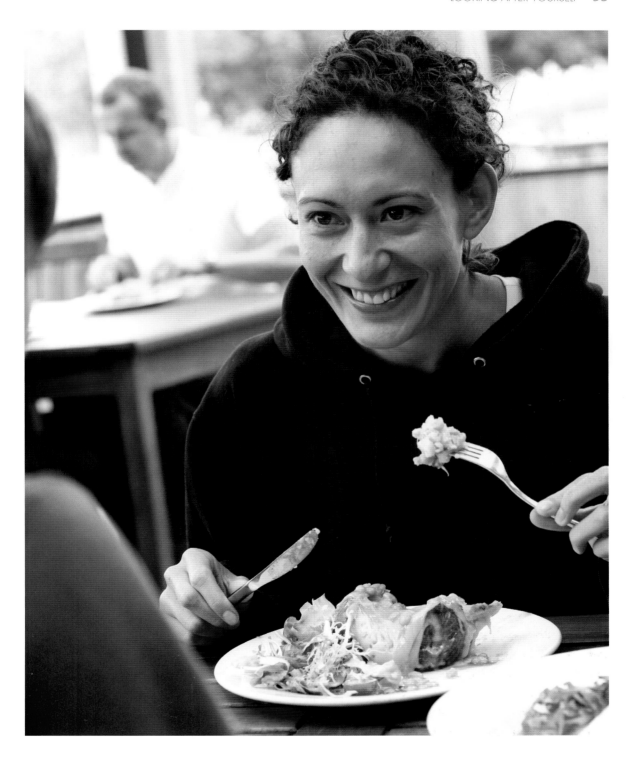

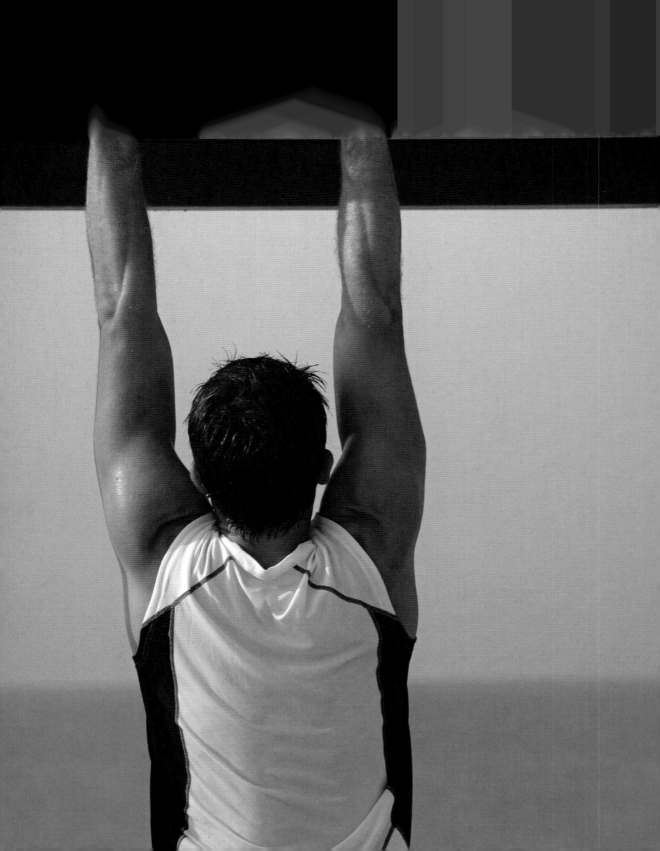

land training:
it's not all about the water

TRAINING ON LAND

Specificity in training is essential to improve your swimming performance—so if you want to improve your front crawl technique and performance, for example, you need to swim front crawl. However, in contrast to this fundamental principle of training is the concept of cross-training—using alternative methods of training to enhance performance in your chosen event.

Training on land in addition to in the water is commonly used by competitive swimmers, and is as relevent for the recreational swimmer. Regular land training will enable you to improve your flexibility, strength and strength endurance, as well as reduce the risk of injury and add variety to your training program.

Flexibility and strength are important elements of swimming performance, as they underlie technical ability and cardiovascular endurance, and reduce the risk of injury. Without flexibility and strength, your endurance capacity would be significantly reduced. In addition to the swimming benefits, flexibility and strength training develop tone in your muscles, giving your body shape and form. So you can swim faster and look great. (Check out the bodies of competitive swimmers!)

I have divided this chapter into four sections, in which you will find exercises for:

- flexibility
- strength
- core stability
- strength endurance

FLEXIBILITY

Poor flexibility is a common reason for finding it difficult to master a swimming technique. Stiffness, particularly around the shoulders and neck, often results in poor technique and will restrict your capacity for improvement. Flexibility of the legs and ankles is also important, particularly for the breast stroke.

Flexibility should be part of your warm-up and cool-down for each of your swimming sessions. In addition, dedicated flexibility sessions are great for improving your range of motion and can really make a difference in the water.

A range of flexibility exercises is set out in this section, many of which you can do any time, anywhere, and at a level appropriate to you.

During these exercises it is important that you move slowly to a position where you first feel the stretch in the target area, then hold that position for thirty seconds. In order to allow the muscles to lengthen, you need to stay as relaxed as possible when stretching. To do this, try focusing on breathing deeply throughout. Never push yourself to a position that causes pain.

Neck

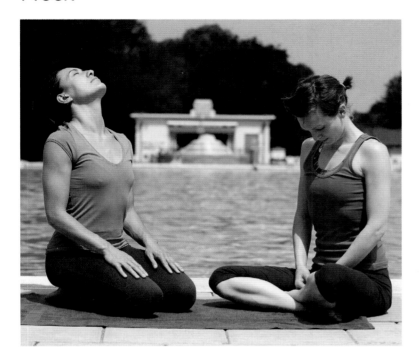

Neck extension

- Sit or stand with your body upright and stable.
- Raise your chin as high as possible, keeping your mouth closed, without leaning back.

Hold for 20–30 seconds.

Neck flexion

- Sit or stand with your body upright and stable.
- Lower your chin to your chest without leaning forward.

Hold for 20–30 seconds.

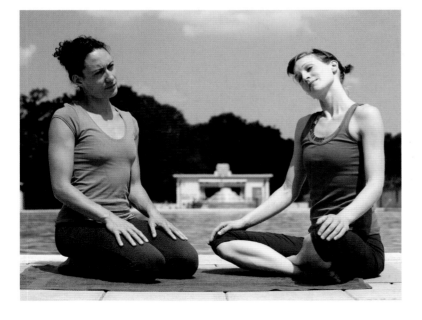

Side neck

- Sit or stand with your body upright and stable.
- Lower your ear toward your shoulder on the same side.

When you feel a stretch, hold for 20–30 seconds. Repeat on the other side.

Chest and arms

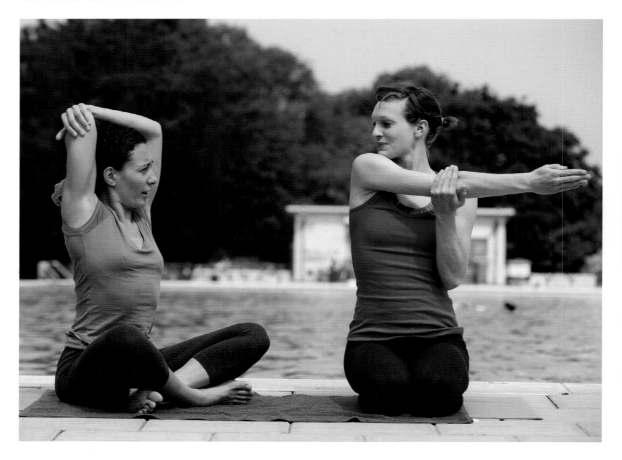

Triceps

- Sit or stand with your body upright and stable.
- Lift one arm above your head and bend it at the elbow with your hand pointing down your back.
- Cup your elbow with the opposite hand and ease the elbow toward your head until you feel a stretch in the back of your upper arm.

Hold for 20–30 seconds. Repeat with the other arm.

Back of shoulder

- Sit or stand with your body upright and stable.
- Bring one arm across your chest toward the opposite shoulder without rotating your upper body.
- Cup your elbow with your hand and pull the arm toward your chest until you feel a stretch in the back of your shoulder.

Hold for 20–30 seconds. Repeat with the other arm.

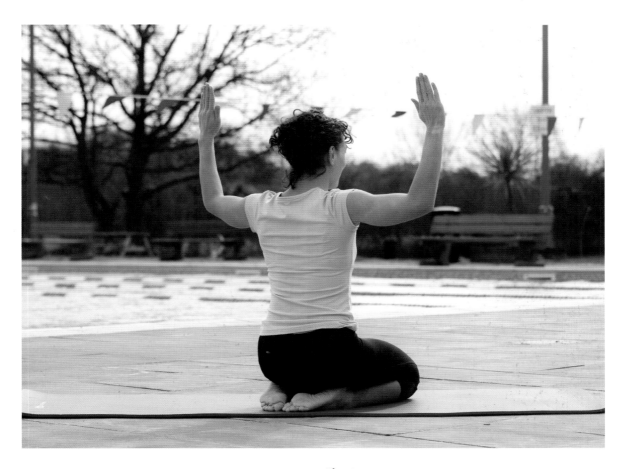

Chest

- Sit or stand with your body upright and stable.
- Bend your arms to 90 degrees and raise them out to the sides until your elbows are at shoulder height.
- Pull your elbows backward and push your chest out until you feel a stretch across your chest.

Hold for 20–30 seconds.

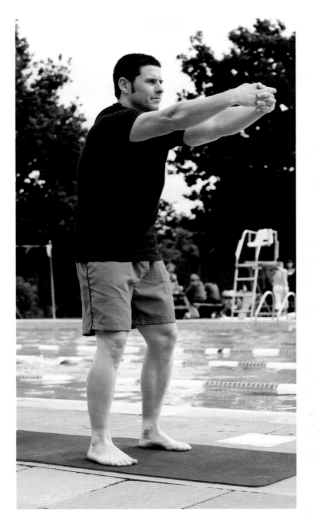

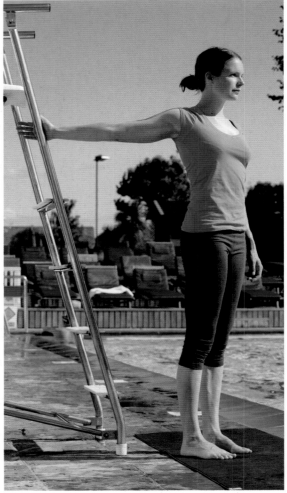

Shoulders

- Stand upright with feet shoulder-width apart and facing forward.
- Interlock your fingers and stretch your arms out in front of you.
- Round your shoulders and push out your shoulder blades.

Hold for 20–30 seconds.

Biceps

- Stand upright next to a wall or door with feet shoulder-width apart, facing forward.
- Place the palm of one hand against the wall at shoulder height.
- Keeping your arm straight, turn your body away from the wall until you feel a stretch along the front of your arm.

Hold for 20–30 seconds. Repeat with the other arm.

Back and side

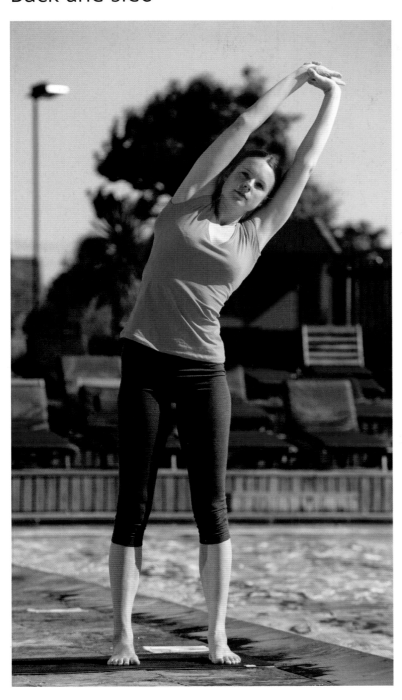

Side bend

- Stand upright with feet shoulder-width apart, facing forward.
- Place your right arm above your head and clasp the wrist with your left hand.
- Lean to your left, without bending forward or backward, until you feel a stretch down your side.

Hold for 20–30 seconds. Repeat with the other side.

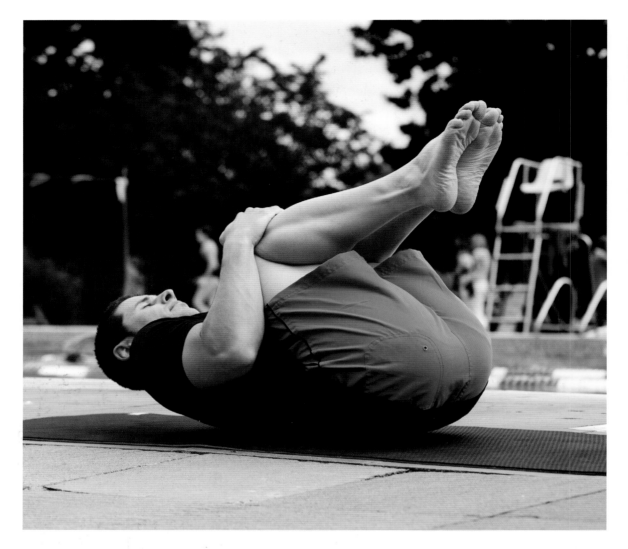

Back

- Lie on your back and bend your knees up toward your chest.
- Place your hands on your knees and pull your knees farther toward your chest.

Hold for 20–30 seconds.

Lower back

- Kneel down on the floor and sit on your heels.
- Rest your body on your thighs.
- Place your forehead on the ground and arms in front of you.

  Relax and hold for 20–30 seconds.

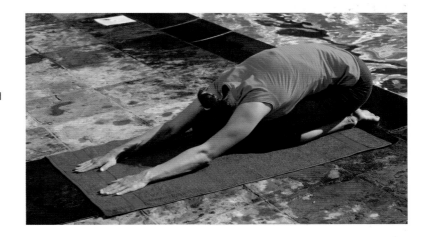

Upper-body stretch

- Kneel down on the floor and sit on your heels.
- Rest your body on your thighs.
- Place your forehead on the ground and have your arms outstretched in front of you.
- Keeping your forehead near to the ground, walk your hands slowly to the left until you feel a stretch along your upper body.

  Relax and hold for 20–30 seconds. Move the right and hold for 20–30 seconds.

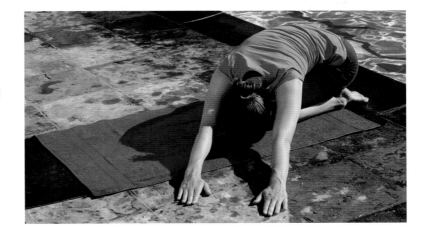

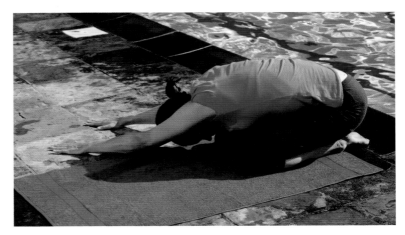

Hips and groin

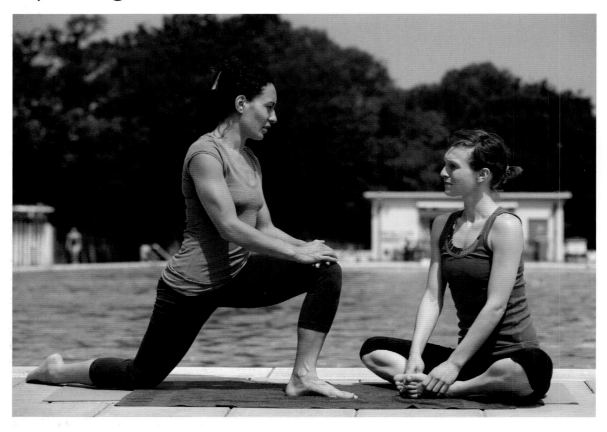

Hip flexor

- From a lunge position, drop your back knee to the floor, well behind your hip (place a cushion under your knee if necessary).
- Place your hands on your knee or on the floor on either side of your foot.
- Move your pelvis forward until your front knee is at 90 degrees and you feel the stretch in the front of your hip joint and thigh.

Hold for 20–30 seconds. Repeat with the other leg.

Groin

- Sitting up with a straight back, place the soles of your feet together.
- Hold your feet with both hands and press your knees to the ground until you feel a stretch.

Hold for 20–30 seconds.

Bum and hip

- Lie on your back with both legs bent.
- Place the ankle of one leg on the knee of the other.
- Place your hands behind the back knee and pull it toward your chest.

Hold for 20–30 seconds. Repeat with the other leg.

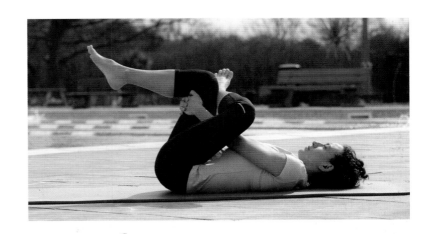

Outer thigh

- Sit on the floor with your legs out straight in front of you.
- Bend your right leg and place the foot over your left leg.
- Rotate your body and place your left arm over the right leg.
- Ease your right knee to the left.

Hold for 20–30 seconds. Repeat with the right leg.

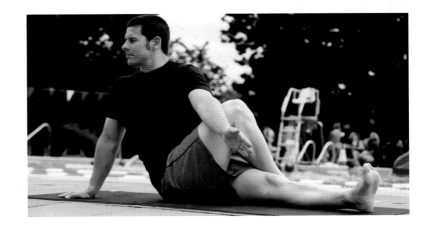

Z-stretch for hips

- Sit on the floor with one leg bent in front of you and one leg bent behind you (making a Z shape).
- Curl your body over your front leg.
- Place your elbows on the ground, keeping your spine as straight as possible.

Hold for 20–30 seconds. Repeat with the other leg.

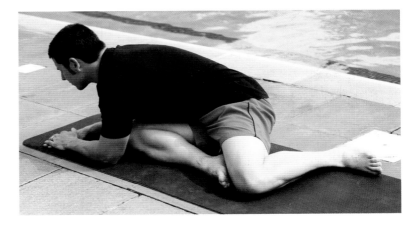

Legs

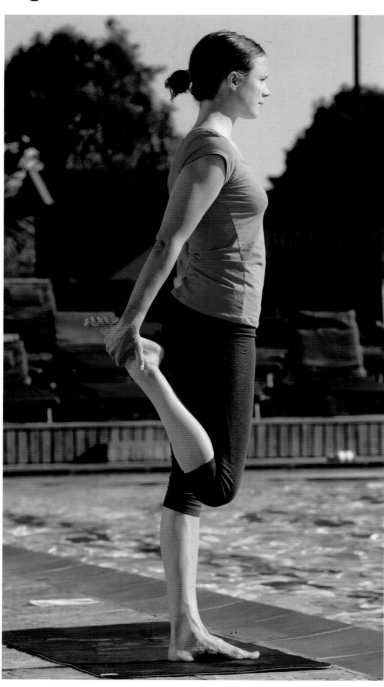

Thigh

- Stand with your body upright and stable.
- Bend one leg and pull the heel toward your bum (hold on to something for stability if needed).
- Keep the shoulders, hips and knees in line.

Hold for 20–30 seconds. Repeat with the other leg.

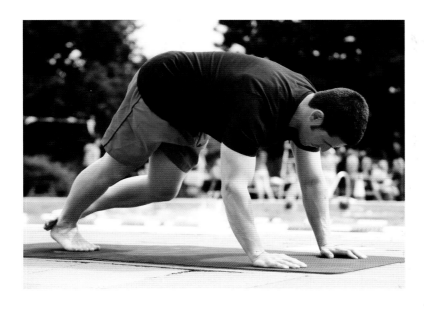

Calf

- With your hands on the ground, shoulder-width apart, stretch your legs out behind you so that the balls of your feet are on the ground.
- Place your left foot over your right ankle.
- Lengthen the right leg and press the heel toward the ground until you feel a stretch down the back of the calf.

Hold for 20–30 seconds. Repeat on the other side.

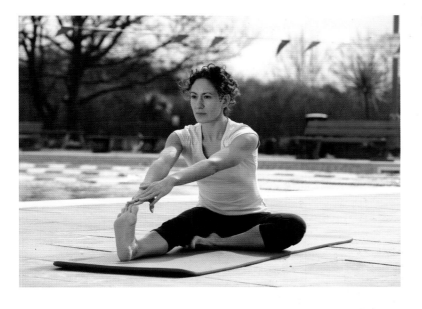

Hamstring

- Sit with your body upright, one leg extended in front of you and the other leg bent bent in front of you.
- Bend forward, reaching for your toes until you feel a stretch along the back of your leg.

Hold for 20–30 seconds. Repeat with the other leg.

STRENGTH

Strength refers to your ability to apply muscular force in order to move an object. It is not only associated with the size of the muscle, but also with the way in which you recruit the muscle (ask it to work). In other words, you can be strong without having big muscles. Given the nature of swimming, upper-body strength is more important than lower-body strength, although the legs and core are crucial for maintaining optimum body position for fast swimming.

In this section you will find a range of exercises that you can use to improve your upper- and lower-body strength. The strength exercises require specialized equipment that is available at most gyms. However, the exercises in the Core Stability and Strength Endurance sections can be done at home (see pages 120–128).

Workouts can be tough and should be done separately from your swimming sessions. Also, make sure you build in enough recovery into your program to avoid injury.

When performing strength exercises you should concentrate on using the full range of motion. In addition, apply force slowly and deliberately, concentrating on correct posture and technique.

Arms

Shoulder press
- Sit directly below the bar with a straight back and your feet flat on the floor.
- With the bar in line with your shoulders slowly extend your arms above your head until straight (avoid locking the elbows).

Slowly return your hands to the starting position and repeat.

Biceps curl
- Stand with a straight back, holding the bar with your palms facing upward.
- Slowly pull your arms upward without using excessive movement of your back.

Slowly return your arms to the starting position and repeat.

HOW MANY REPS SHOULD I DO?

If you are new to these exercises, start off with a light weight and three sets of ten repetitions. Only increase the weight when you are able to complete the third set of ten repetitions easily. If you are unsure, ask a personal trainer for advice; it is always better to be safe than sorry!

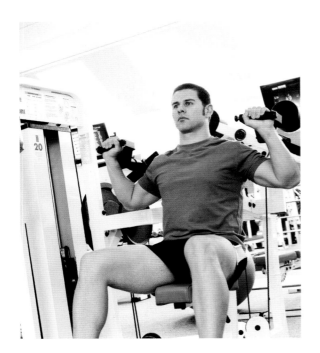

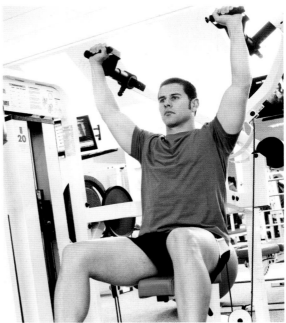

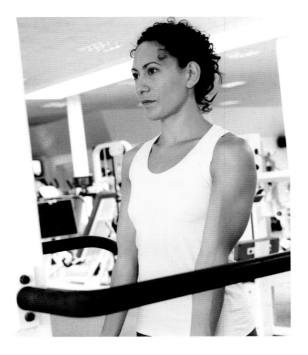

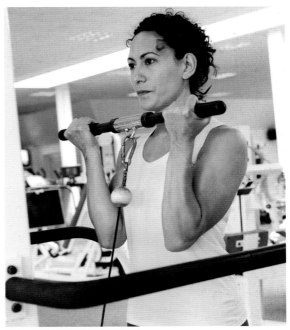

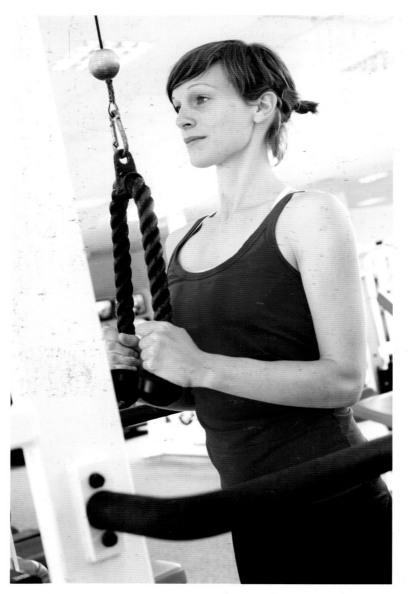

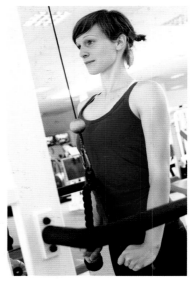

Triceps extension

- Stand with a straight back holding the ropes in front of you.
- Slowly extend your arms downward until they are straight, without using excessive movement of your back (avoid locking the arms).

Slowly return your arms to the starting position and repeat.

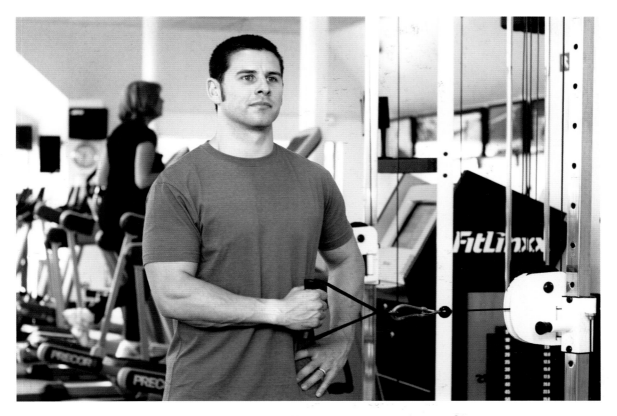

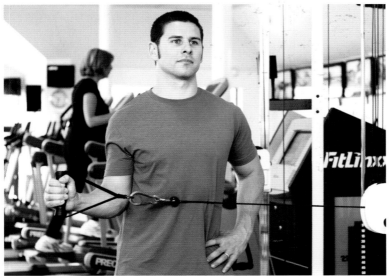

External rotation

- Stand upright with your feet sideways on to the pulley, shoulder-width apart.
- With the pulley set at a height corresponding to the height of your hand when the elbow is flexed at 90 degrees, slowly rotate your arm outward, keeping your elbow touching your side and without using excessive movement of your back.

Slowly return your arms to the starting position and repeat.

Chest and back

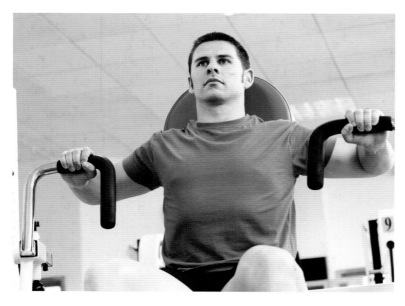

Bench press

- Sit with the bar in line with your chest and your feet flat on the floor.
- Slowly extend your arms directly forward until they are straight (avoid locking the elbows).

Slowly return your hands to the starting position and repeat.

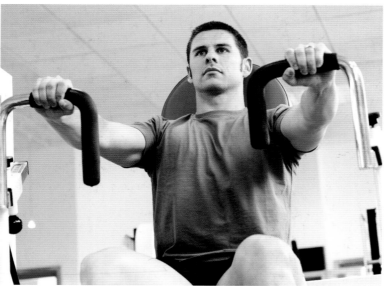

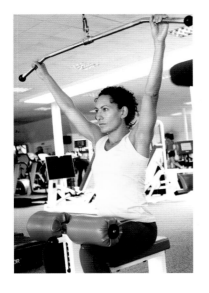 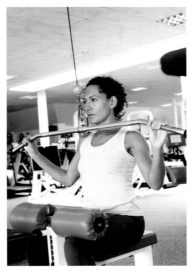

Lat pull-down

- Sit directly below the bar with a straight back and your feet flat on the floor.
- With the bar in line with your shoulders and your arms fully extended, slowly pull your arms down to your chest without using excessive movement of your back.

Slowly return your hands to the starting position and repeat.

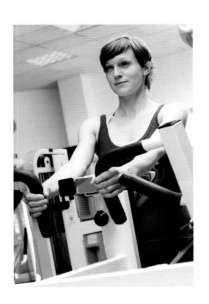 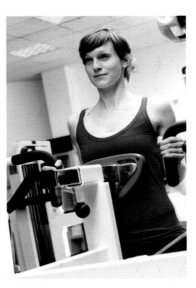

Standing rowing

- Stand with your back straight, holding the bars in front of you with your arms fully extended.
- Slowly pull your hands toward your chest without using excessive movement of your back.

Slowly return your hands to the starting position and repeat.

Hips

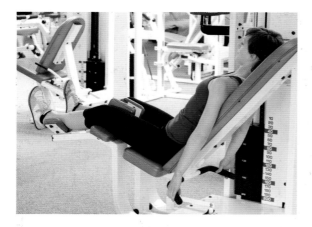

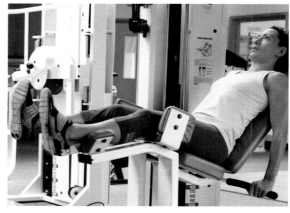

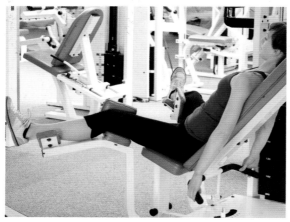

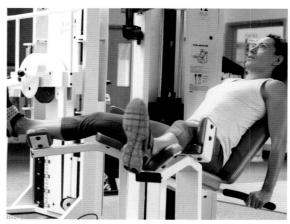

Inner hip

- Sit with your inner thighs pressed against the cushioned pads.
- Release the brake and slowly open your legs to a comfortable (but challenging) position, holding on to the handles to avoid excessive movement of the body.

Slowly return your legs to the starting position and repeat.

Outer hip

- Sit with your outer thighs pressed against the cushioned pads.
- Release the brake and slowly open your legs to a comfortable (but challenging) position, holding on to the handles to avoid excessive movement of the body.

Slowly return your legs to the starting position and repeat.

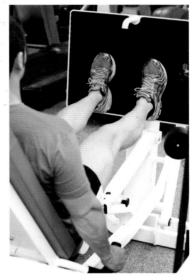

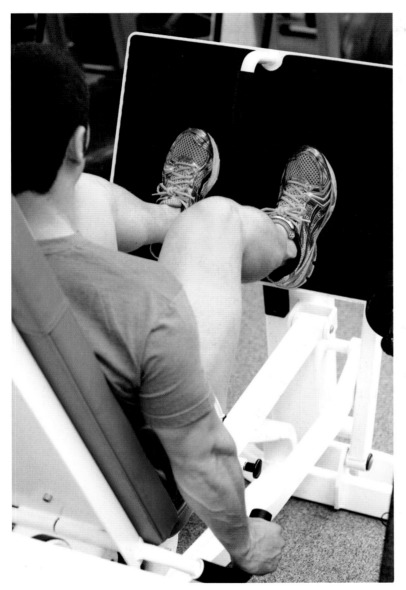

Hack squat

- Sit with your feet on the platform, knees flexed at around 90 degrees.
- Slowly extend your legs (avoid locking the knees), holding on to the handles to avoid excessive movement of the body.

Slowly return your legs to the starting position and repeat.

Legs

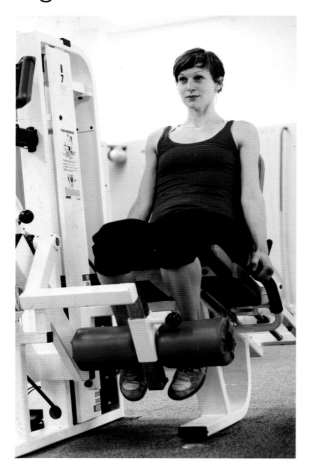 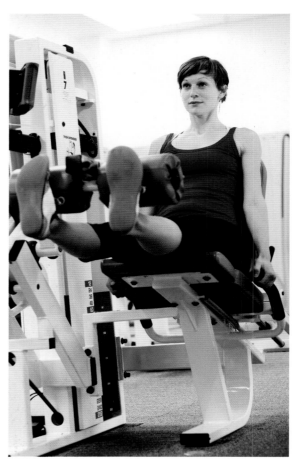

Leg extension

- Sit with your feet placed under the cushioned pad and knees flexed.
- Slowly extend your legs (avoid locking the knees), holding on to the handles to avoid excessive movement of the body.

Slowly return your legs to the starting position and repeat.

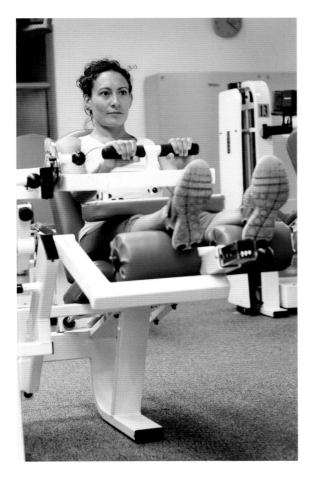 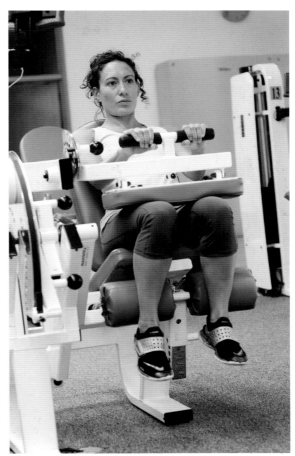

Leg curl

- Sit with your legs fully extended on top of the cushioned pad (avoid locking the knees).
- Slowly flex your legs to around 90 degrees, holding on to the handles to avoid excessive movement of the body.

Slowly return your legs to the starting position and repeat.

CORE STABILITY EXERCISES

Having strong core muscles (tummy, bottom, and lower back) is crucial for swimming because it will enable you to maintain a streamlined body position, as well as help you control the movement of your arms and legs.

Having a strong core also plays an important part in reducing back pain and other injuries that are common in swimmers. The following section demonstrates a range of exercises that will help you develop your core stability.

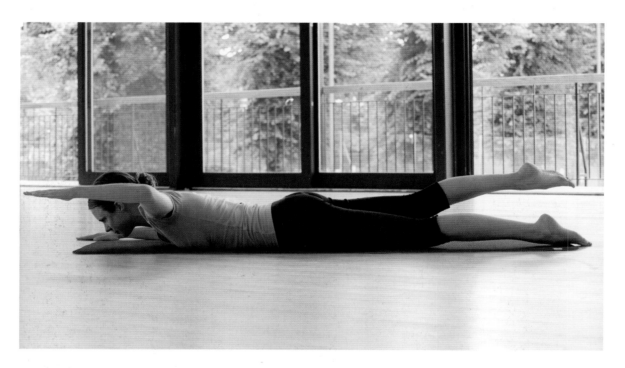

Lower back and core

- Lie facedown with your arms out to the sides, elbows bent to 90 degrees and feet hip-width apart.
- Lift your left arm and right leg simultaneously and hold for 5 seconds.
- Return to the start position.
- Lift your right arm and left leg simultaneously and hold for 5 seconds.

- Return to the start position.

  Repeat the cycle 10 times.

  (Note: you need to think about length rather than height here—stretch out the limbs.)

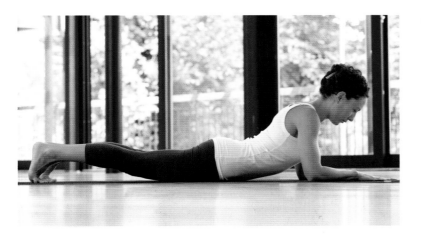

Plank

- Lie on your stomach with your forearms on the ground, palms facing down and level with the top of your head.
- Raise yourself onto your forearms and the balls of your feet, making a straight line between your heel, hips, and shoulders.

Hold for 20 seconds. Relax and repeat 3 times.

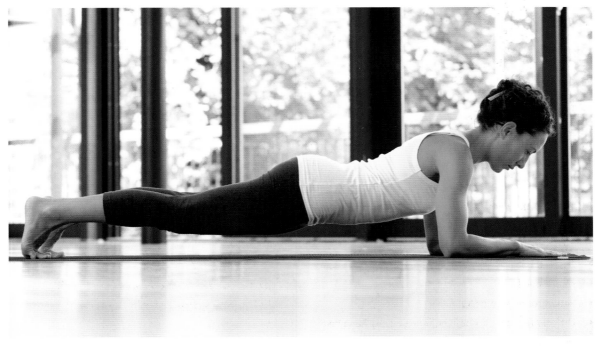

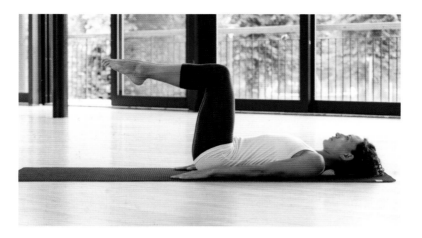

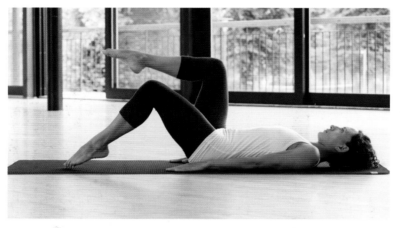

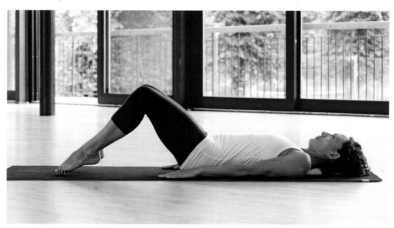

Toe touch

- Lie on your back with your arms by your sides.
- Pull your knees up and hold them in the air, making 90-degree angles at your hips and knees.
- Engage your core (inner stomach muscles) and lower one foot to the floor, touching the toe lightly on the ground before returning to the start position.

Repeat with the other leg. Repeat the cycle 10 times.

MAKE IT HARDER

- Engage your core (inner stomach muscles) and lower both feet to the floor, touching the toes lightly on the floor before returning to the start position.

Repeat 20 times.

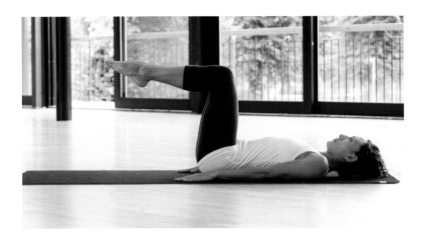

Leg lower

- Lie on your back with your arms by your sides.
- Pull your knees up and hold them in the air, making 90 degree angles at your hips and knees.
- Without arching your back, lower your toes toward the floor and straighten your legs.

Return to the start position.
Repeat 10 times.

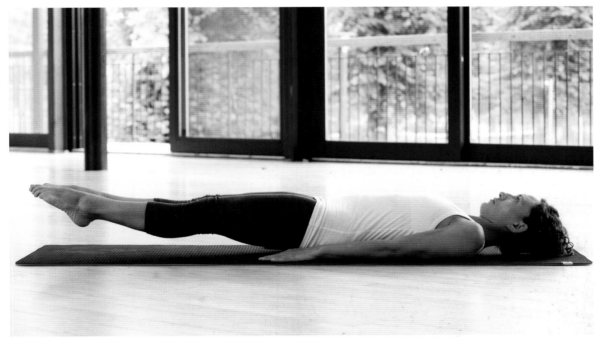

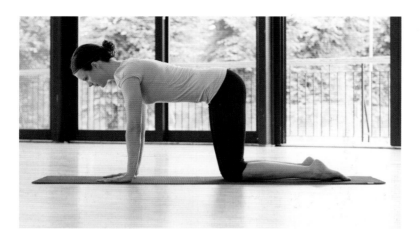

Cat

- Begin on all fours with your weight evenly distributed between your hands and knees and your back long and straight.
- Engage all of the muscles surrounding your abdomen and, without collapsing your arms, extend your left leg directly backward and your right arm directly forward.
- Hold for 5 seconds.
- Return to the start position.
- Repeat with the right leg and left arm.

Relax and repeat the cycle 5 times.

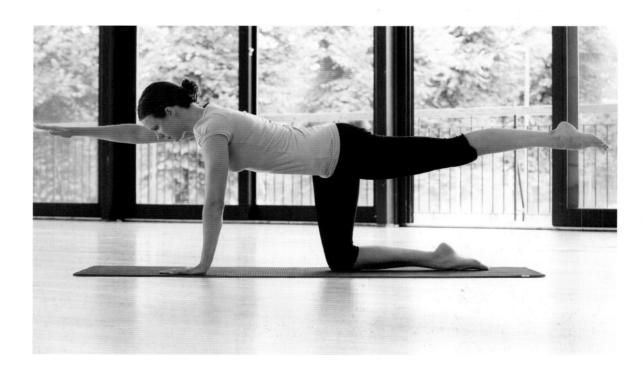

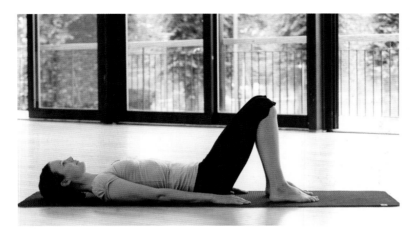

Shoulder bridge

- Lie on your back, hands by your sides and knees bent with feet shoulder-width apart.
- Breathe in and roll your hips to the ceiling until you are resting on your shoulders with a straight line from shoulders to hips to knees.
- In that position, maintaining level knees, extend one leg and hold for 10 seconds.
- Return to the start position and repeat with the other leg.

Relax and repeat the cycle 5 times.

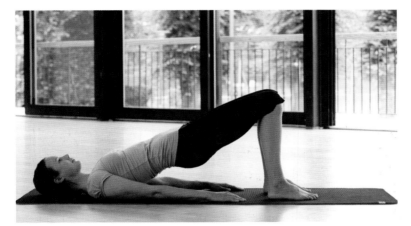

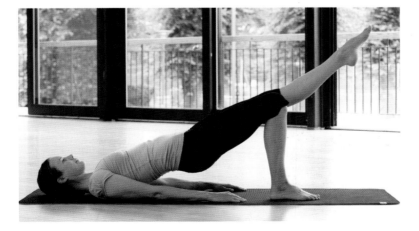

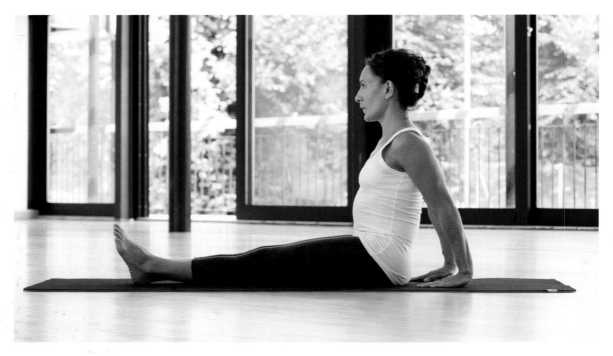

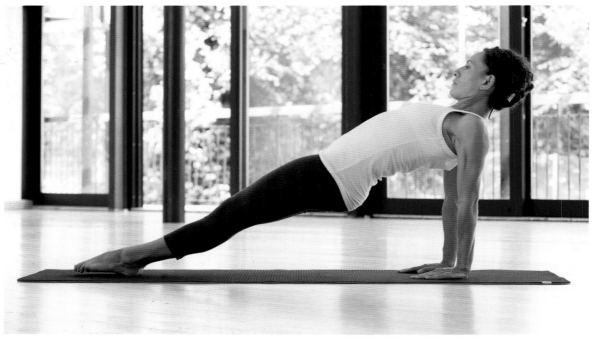

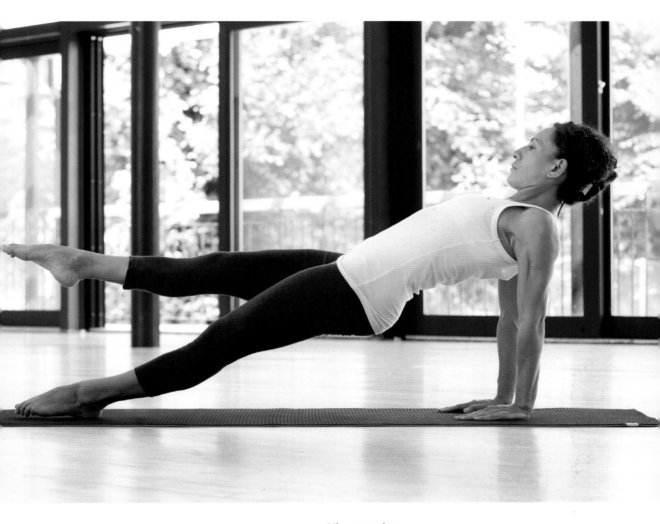

Hip extension

- Sit with your legs extended in front of you and your hands on the floor behind you.
- Lift your hips to the ceiling, making a straight line from shoulders to hips to ankles.
- In that position, lift one leg to the same height as your hip and hold for 10 seconds.
- Repeat with your other leg.

Return to the start position and repeat 3 times.

STRENGTH ENDURANCE

Strength endurance refers to your ability to maintain strength exercises over time. This type of fitness is very important for swimming and although swimming itself will improve your strength endurance, land-based strength endurance provides a great alternative and can make a refreshing change.

Circuit training

Circuits are one of the best ways to improve strength endurance. They are composed of a number of specific exercises that are performed at a hard level with relatively short recoveries in between. You can mix and match exercises to add variety to sessions as well as target particular muscle groups.

If you are training in the gym you could use any of the strength exercises described in this chapter (see pages 110–119). Alternatively, you could design a circuit that doesn't use machines so that you can do it at home, in the park, or even in the office! Possible exercises you could include are press-ups, sit-ups, skipping, stair-climbing, running, and any of the core stability exercises in this chapter (see pages 120–127).

There are several formats that you can use with circuits. You can select a large number of different exercises (e.g. fifteen) and run through them sequentially, performing each one for a specified period (e.g. thirty seconds) or number of repetitions (e.g. twenty), with a short recovery (e.g. thirty seconds). Alternatively, you could select a smaller number of exercises (three to five) and repeat the circuit three times with short recoveries in between.

The difficulty of circuits can be upped in a number of other ways. You can add additional exercises, increase how hard/fast you are performing each exercise, or increase the number of times you complete the circuit. In addition, rather than having inactive rest between the exercises, you could perform easy to medium-level aerobic exercise, such as jogging or skipping—this can make circuits really tough!

To ease the boredom of exercising alone, or to give yourself a new challenge, why not join a circuit class? Let someone else motivate you while you grunt and sweat! As with strength sessions, circuits can be tough and it is best to do them separately from your swimming session to avoid excessive tiredness. It is also advisable to stretch before and after workouts to avoid possible injury.

RIGHT: Skip to it—land training is great for strength endurance and adds variety to your workout.

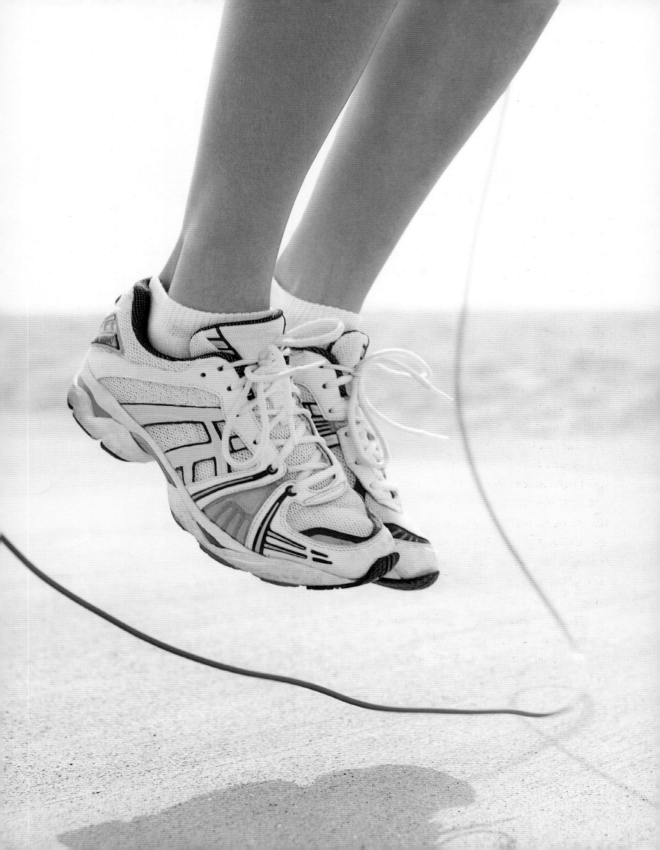

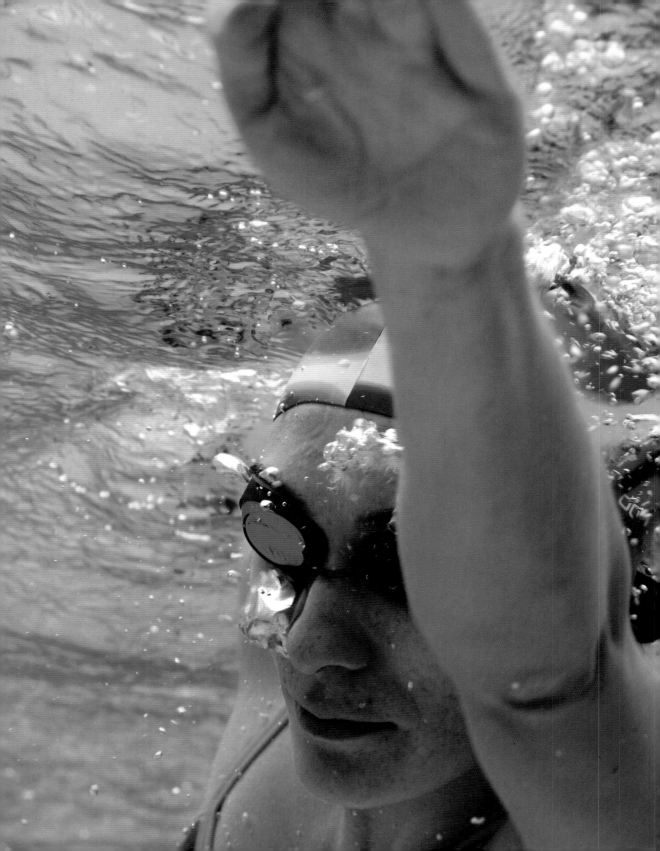

training
programs

SWIMMING PROGRAMS

This chapter provides you with examples of programs for beginner, intermediate, and advanced swimmers. Each program is presented over a six-week period to demonstrate how you can boost your swimming volume by increasing how long you swim for, how hard you swim, and how many sessions you do per week. Note that the programs are designed for 20 meter or 25 meter swimming pools—for longer pools, reduce the number of lengths or the number of swims to maintain the same distance.

Each swimming session is made up of episodes or blocks of swimming with various strokes, including front crawl, breast stroke, back stroke, and butterfly as well as kicking only and pulling (arms only) lengths. The programs outline how far to swim with a given stroke, how hard (indicated by "easy," "medium" or "hard"), and the amount of recovery time allowed between blocks. You should try to take your rest in the shallow end to allow you to recover fully. When your recovery period is not in shallow water, hold on to the side or the lane rope to make sure you are getting as much rest as possible.

These programs are simply a guide, and you should tailor them to your own ability and goals. For example, if you are a beginner or you're returning to swimming after a long time out of the water you need not necessarily aim for three to four sessions per week—one may be enough. It is also possible to keep the same total of lengths done in a week, but vary the number of sessions it is reached in, increasing or decreasing as necessary.

You can monitor how much swimming you are doing in each session and over a week (or longer) by using the simple formula on page 56. On the opposite page is a example table

Elements to include in your program:

- **Front crawl**
- **Breast stroke**
- **Back stroke**
- **Butterfly**
- **Kicking (using legs only)**
- **Pulling (using arms only)**

to demonstrate how a beginner would score their training sessions over a week.

Trying to remember your swimming session can be difficult, so why not photocopy or print your program and laminate it to stop it from disintegrating on the poolside, or simply use a zip-top sandwich bag to keep it dry.

See also:

- Chapter 2, pages 27–49 for swimming technique.
- Chapter 3, pages 51–65 for information on structuring and monitoring your swimming sessions.
- Chapter 4, pages 68–77 for ways to keep yourself motivated.

Scoring a week's training:

Monday	Rest	
Tuesday	• 5 lengths front crawl easy • 10 x 1 length front crawl hard (30 seconds recovery between each) • 5 lengths front crawl easy	5 x 1 = 5 points 10 x 3 = 30 points 5 x 1 = 5 points **SESSION TOTAL = 40 points**
Wednesday	Rest	
Thursday	Rest	
Friday	• 5 lengths breast stroke easy • 2 x 5 lengths front crawl hard (1 minute recovery between each set) • 5 lengths front crawl easy	5 x 1 = 5 points 10 x 3 = 30 points 5 x 1 = 5 points **SESSION TOTAL = 40 points**
Saturday	Rest	
Sunday	• 5 lengths front crawl easy • 10 lengths breast stroke hard • 5 lengths front crawl kick	5 x 1 = 5 points 10 x 3 = 30 points 5 x 1 = 5 points **SESSION TOTAL = 40 points**

WEEK TOTAL = 120 POINTS

WEEK 1	BEGINNER (15–20 lengths)	INTERMEDIATE (20–30 lengths)	ADVANCED (50–60 lengths)

Monday	Rest	• 10 lengths front crawl easy
		• 5 x 1 length front crawl hard
		  (30 seconds recovery between each)
		• 5 x 1 length breast stroke hard
		  (30 seconds recovery between each)
			• 10 lengths front crawl easy
			• 2 x 10 lengths front crawl hard
			  (30 seconds recovery after each set)
			• 10 lengths front crawl pulling medium
			• 5 x 1 length front crawl kick
			  (30 seconds recovery between each)
			• 10 lengths front crawl easy

Tuesday	• 5 lengths front crawl easy
	• 10 x 1 length front crawl hard
	  (30 seconds recovery between each)
	• 5 lengths front crawl easy
		Rest	• 10 lengths front crawl
			• 2 x 10 lengths front crawl hard
			  (30 seconds recovery after each set)
			• 2 x 2 lengths back stroke hard
			  (15 seconds recovery after each set)
			• 2 x 2 lengths breast stroke hard
			  (15 seconds recovery after each set)
			• 2 x 1 length butterfly hard
			  (30 seconds recovery between each)
			• 10 lengths front crawl easy

Wednesday	Rest	• 5 lengths front crawl easy
		• 2 x 5 lengths front crawl hard
		  (1 minute recovery after each set)
		• 2 x 5 lengths breast stroke hard
		  (1 minute recovery after each set)
		• 5 lengths back stroke easy
			Rest

Thursday	Rest	• 10 lengths front crawl easy
		• 5 x 1 length breast stroke kick
		  (30 seconds recovery between each)
		• 5 x 1 length front crawl kick
		  (30 seconds recovery between each)
		• 10 lengths front crawl easy
			• 10 lengths front crawl easy
			• 3 x 10 lengths front crawl pulling hard
			  (30 seconds recovery after each set)
			• 10 x 1 length front crawl kicking
			  (30 seconds recovery between each)
			• 10 lengths front crawl easy

Friday	• 5 lengths breast stroke easy • 5 lengths front crawl hard • 5 lengths front crawl medium • 5 lengths front crawl easy	Rest	• 25 lengths front crawl medium • 15 lengths back stroke hard • 10 lengths breast stroke hard • 5 x 2 lengths butterfly hard (15 seconds recovery after each set)
Saturday	Rest	• 3 x 10 lengths front crawl medium (1 minute recovery after each set)	Rest
Sunday	• 5 lengths front crawl • 10 lengths breast stroke hard • 5 lengths front crawl kick	Rest	• 3 x 20 lengths front crawl medium (1 minute recovery after each set)

WEEK 2	BEGINNER (20 lengths)	INTERMEDIATE (30–40 lengths)	ADVANCED (60–70 lengths)
Monday	• 20 lengths front crawl medium	Rest	• 10 lengths front crawl easy • 3 x 5 lengths breast stroke pulling (30 seconds recovery after each set) • 5 x 2 lengths breast stroke kick (30 seconds recovery after each set) • 3 x 5 lengths breast stroke hard (1 minute recovery after each set) • 10 lengths front crawl
Tuesday	Rest	• 10 lengths front crawl easy • 10 x 2 lengths front crawl hard (30 seconds recovery after each set) • 10 lengths breast stroke kick	• 5 lengths front crawl easy • 30 lengths front crawl hard • 20 lengths front crawl pull hard • 10 lengths front crawl kick hard • 5 lengths front crawl easy
Wednesday	Rest	Rest	Rest
Thursday	• 5 lengths front crawl easy • 5 lengths breast stroke hard • 5 lengths back stroke hard • 5 lengths front crawl easy	• 10 lengths front crawl easy • 5 x 2 lengths front crawl hard (1 minute recovery after each set) • 5 x 2 lengths breast stroke hard (30 seconds recovery after each set) • 5 x 1 length back stroke hard (30 seconds recovery between each) • 5 lengths front crawl easy	• 10 lengths front crawl • 4 x 5 lengths front crawl hard (30 seconds recovery after each set) • 4 x 5 lengths back stroke hard (30 seconds recovery after each set) • 2 x 5 lengths breast stroke hard (30 seconds recovery after each set) • 5 x 1 length butterfly hard (30 seconds recovery between each) • 5 lengths front crawl easy
Friday	Rest	• 10 lengths front crawl easy • 5 lengths front crawl pulling hard • 5 lengths front crawl kick hard • 5 lengths front crawl pulling hard • 5 lengths front crawl easy	• 10 lengths front crawl easy • 10 x 4 lengths front crawl hard (30 seconds recovery after each set) • 10 x 1 length front crawl hard (30 seconds recovery between each) • 10 lengths front crawl easy
Saturday	• 5 lengths front crawl easy • 5 x 1 length front crawl hard (30 seconds recovery between each) • 5 x 1 length back stroke hard (30 seconds recovery between each) • 5 lengths front crawl easy	Rest	• 3 x 20 lengths front crawl medium (1 minute recovery after each set)
Sunday	• 20 lengths front crawl medium	• 2 x 20 lengths front crawl medium (1 minute recovery after each set)	Rest

WEEK 3	BEGINNER (20–30 lengths)	INTERMEDIATE (50 lengths)	ADVANCED (60–80 lengths)
Monday	Rest	• 20 lengths front crawl easy • 5 x 2 lengths front crawl hard (30 seconds recovery after each set) • 5 x 2 lengths breast stroke hard (30 seconds recovery after each set) • 10 lengths front crawl easy	• 10 lengths front crawl easy • 3 x 10 lengths front crawl medium (30 seconds recovery after each set) • 10 lengths front crawl pulling medium • 5 x 1 length butterfly hard (30 seconds recovery between each) • 10 lengths front crawl easy
Tuesday	• 5 lengths front crawl easy • 10 x 1 length front crawl hard (30 seconds recovery between each) • 5 lengths front crawl easy	Rest	• 5 lengths front crawl easy • 3 x 10 lengths front crawl medium (30 seconds recovery after each set) • 5 x 3 lengths back stroke hard (15 seconds recovery after each set) • 5 x 3 lengths breast stroke hard (15 seconds recovery after each set) • 5 x 1 length butterfly hard (30 seconds recovery between each) • 5 lengths front crawl easy
Wednesday	Rest	• 10 lengths front crawl easy • 4 x 5 lengths front crawl hard (1 minute recovery after each set) • 5 lengths breast stroke kick • 5 lengths back stroke kick • 10 lengths front crawl easy	Rest
Thursday	Rest	• 10 lengths front crawl easy • 2 x 5 lengths breast stroke hard (30 seconds recovery after each set) • 2 x 5 lengths back stroke hard (30 seconds recovery after each set) • 2 x 5 lengths front crawl hard (30 seconds recovery after each set) • 10 lengths front crawl	• 10 lengths front crawl easy • 5 x 5 lengths front crawl hard (30 seconds recovery between each) • 10 lengths front crawl kick • 10 x 1 length front crawl hard (30 seconds recovery between each) • 10 lengths front crawl easy
Friday	• 5 lengths breast stroke easy • 5 lengths front crawl hard • 5 x 1 length front crawl hard (30 seconds recovery between each) • 5 lengths front crawl hard • 5 lengths breast stroke	Rest	• 30 lengths front crawl medium • 20 lengths back stroke medium • 10 lengths breast stroke hard • 5 x 2 lengths butterfly hard (15 seconds recovery after each set)
Saturday	Rest	• 2 x 25 lengths front crawl medium (1 minute recovery after each set)	Rest
Sunday	• 10 lengths front crawl medium • 10 lengths breast stroke medium • 5 lengths front crawl hard • 5 lengths breast stroke hard	Rest	• 2 x 30 lengths front crawl medium (1 minute recovery after each set)

WEEK 4	BEGINNER (30 lengths)	INTERMEDIATE (50–60 lengths)	ADVANCED (80–90 lengths)
Monday	• 5 lengths front crawl medium • 5 lengths back stroke medium • 5 lengths breast stroke medium • 10 x 1 length front crawl hard (30 seconds recovery between each) • 5 lengths front crawl easy	Rest	• 10 lengths front crawl easy • 4 x 10 lengths front crawl hard (30 seconds recovery after each set) • 5 x 2 lengths front crawl hard (30 seconds recovery after each set) • 10 x 1 length front crawl hard (1 minute recovery between each) • 10 lengths front crawl easy
Tuesday	Rest	• 10 lengths front crawl easy • 10 x 4 lengths front crawl hard (30 seconds recovery after each set) • 10 lengths front crawl easy	• 10 lengths front crawl easy • 20 lengths front crawl pulling hard • 20 lengths breast stroke pulling hard • 20 lengths back stroke pulling hard • 10 lengths front crawl easy
Wednesday	Rest	Rest	Rest
Thursday	• 5 lengths front crawl easy • 10 lengths breast stroke pulling • 10 lengths breast stroke kick • 5 lengths breast stroke easy	• 10 lengths front crawl easy • 5 x 2 lengths front crawl hard (1 minute recovery after each set) • 5 x 2 lengths breast stroke hard (30 seconds recovery after each set) • 5 x 1 length back stroke hard (30 seconds recovery between each) • 5 x 1 length butterfly hard (30 seconds recovery between each) • 10 lengths front crawl easy	• 10 lengths front crawl easy • 5 x 10 lengths front crawl medium (30 seconds recovery after each set) • 5 x 1 length back stroke hard (30 seconds recovery between each) • 5 x 1 length breast stroke hard (30 seconds recovery between each) • 5 x 1 length butterfly hard (30 seconds recovery between each) • 10 lengths front crawl easy
Friday	Rest	• 10 lengths front crawl easy • 4 x 10 lengths front crawl hard (1 minute recovery after each set) • 10 lengths front crawl easy	• 5 lengths front crawl easy • 20 x 4 lengths front crawl hard (30 seconds recovery after each set) • 5 lengths front crawl easy
Saturday	• 5 lengths front crawl easy • 5 x 2 lengths front crawl hard (30 seconds recovery after each set) • 5 x 2 lengths front crawl kick (30 seconds recovery after each set) • 5 lengths front crawl easy	Rest	• 90 lengths front crawl medium
Sunday	• 30 lengths front crawl medium	• 50 lengths front crawl medium	Rest

WEEK 5	BEGINNER (30–40 lengths)	INTERMEDIATE (60 lengths)	ADVANCED (80–100 lengths)
Monday	Rest	• 5 lengths front crawl easy • 10 x 4 lengths front crawl medium (30 seconds recovery after each set) • 10 x 1 length breast stroke hard (30 seconds recovery between each) • 5 lengths front crawl easy	• 10 lengths front crawl easy • 4 x 20 lengths front crawl hard (1 minute recovery after each set) • 10 lengths front crawl pulling medium
Tuesday	• 10 lengths front crawl easy • 5 x 2 lengths front crawl hard (30 seconds recovery after each set) • 5 x 1 length breast stroke hard (30 seconds recovery between each) • 5 x 1 length front crawl hard (30 seconds recovery between each) • 10 lengths front crawl easy	Rest	• 10 lengths front crawl easy • 10 x 4 lengths front crawl hard (30 seconds recovery after each set) • 10 x 2 lengths back stroke (15 seconds recovery after each set) • 10 x 1 length breast stroke hard (15 second recovery between each) • 10 x 1 length butterfly medium (15 second recovery between each) • 10 lengths front crawl easy
Wednesday	Rest	• 10 lengths front crawl easy • 20 lengths front crawl pulling hard • 15 lengths breast stroke kick • 10 lengths back stroke kick • 5 lengths front crawl easy	Rest
Thursday	• 30 lengths front crawl medium	• 10 lengths front crawl easy • 2 x 5 lengths breast stroke hard (30 seconds recovery after each set) • 5 x 2 lengths back stroke hard (15 seconds recovery after each set) • 20 x 1 length front crawl hard (15 seconds recovery between each) • 10 lengths front crawl easy	• 10 lengths front crawl easy • 20 lengths front crawl pulling hard • 20 x 1 length front crawl kick hard (15 seconds recovery between each) • 10 x 2 length front crawl hard (15 seconds recovery after each set) • 10 lengths front crawl easy
Friday	• 10 lengths front crawl easy • 10 lengths front crawl pulling hard • 5 x 2 lengths front crawl kick (30 seconds recovery after each set) • 5 x 1 length back stroke (30 seconds recovery between each) • 5 lengths front crawl easy	Rest	• 10 lengths front crawl easy • 2 x 5 lengths butterfly medium (30 seconds recovery after each set) • 2 x 10 lengths breast stroke hard (30 seconds recovery after each set) • 2 x 10 lengths back stroke hard (30 seconds recovery after each set) • 2 x 10 lengths front crawl hard (30 seconds recovery after each set) • 10 lengths front crawl easy
Saturday	Rest	Rest	Rest
Sunday	• 10 lengths front crawl easy • 5 lengths front crawl pulling medium • 5 lengths back stroke hard • 5 lengths breast stroke kick hard • 10 lengths front crawl easy	• 2 x 30 lengths front crawl medium (1 minute recovery after each set)	• 3 x 30 lengths front crawl medium (1 minute recovery after each set)

WEEK 6	BEGINNER (30–40 lengths)	INTERMEDIATE (50–60 lengths)	ADVANCED (100–110 lengths)
Monday	• 5 lengths front crawl easy • 6 x 4 lengths front crawl (30 seconds recovery after each set) • 5 lengths front crawl easy	Rest	• 10 lengths front crawl easy • 30 lengths front crawl pulling hard • 20 lengths front crawl kick • 30 lengths front crawl hard • 10 lengths front crawl easy

Tuesday	Rest	• 10 lengths front crawl easy
		• 10 x 4 lengths front crawl hard
		  (30 seconds recovery after each set)
		• 10 lengths front crawl easy
			• 10 lengths front crawl easy
			• 10 x 4 lengths front crawl
			  (30 seconds recovery after each set)
			• 5 x 4 lengths back stroke
			  (30 seconds recovery after each set)
			• 5 x 4 lengths breast stroke
			  (30 seconds recovery after each set)
			• 5 x 2 lengths butterfly
			  (40 seconds recovery after each set)
			• 10 lengths front crawl easy

Wednesday	• 5 lengths front crawl easy
	• 10 x 1 length front crawl hard
	  (30 seconds recovery between each)
	• 5 x 1 length breast stroke hard
	  (30 seconds recovery between each)
	• 5 x 1 length back stroke hard
	  (30 seconds recovery between each)
	• 5 lengths front crawl easy
		• 5 lengths front crawl easy
		• 2 x 10 lengths front crawl pulling
		  (1 minute recovery after each set)
		• 2 x 5 lengths front crawl kick
		  (30 seconds recovery after each set)
		• 20 lengths front crawl medium
		  (1 minute recovery after each set)
		• 5 lengths front crawl
			Rest

Thursday	• Rest	• 10 lengths front crawl easy
		• 2 x 5 lengths breast stroke
		  (30 seconds recovery after each set)
		• 2 x 5 lengths back stroke
		  (30 seconds recovery after each set)
		• 2 x 5 lengths front crawl
		  (30 seconds recovery after each set)
		• 10 lengths front crawl easy
			• 10 lengths front crawl easy
			• 20 x 4 lengths front crawl
			  (30 seconds recovery after each set)
			• 10 lengths front crawl easy

Friday	• 10 lengths front crawl easy
	• 5 lengths front crawl pulling hard
	• 5 lengths front crawl kick hard
	• 5 lengths breast stroke pulling hard
	• 5 lengths breast stroke kick hard
	• 10 lengths front crawl easy
		Rest	• 20 lengths front crawl easy
			• 10 x 4 lengths back stroke
			  (30 seconds recovery after each set)
			• 10 x 2 lengths breast stroke
			  (15 seconds recovery after each set)
			• 10 x 1 length butterfly
			  (15 seconds recovery between each)
			• 20 lengths front crawl easy

Saturday	• 10 lengths front crawl medium
	• 10 lengths breast stroke medium
	• 10 lengths back stroke medium
	• 10 lengths front crawl medium
		• 2 x 10 lengths front crawl medium
		  (1 minute recovery after each set)
		• 2 x 10 lengths breast stroke medium
		  (1 minute recovery after each set)
		• 2 x 10 lengths breast stroke medium
		  (1 minute recovery after each set)
			• 100 lengths front crawl medium

Sunday	• 40 lengths front crawl medium	• 60 lengths front crawl medium	Rest

RESOURCES

Swimming Organisations

U.S. MASTERS SWIMMING
655 North Tamiami Trail
Sarasota, FL 34236
800-550-SWIM (7946)
www.usms.org/

USA SWIMMING
USA Swimming National Office
1 Olympic Plaza
Colorado Springs, CO 80909
719-866-4578
www.usaswimming.org/
DesktopDefault.aspx

SWIMMING CANADA
Swimming Canada National Office
2445 St-Laurent Boulevard
Suite B140
Ottawa, ON K1G 6C3
613-260-1348
www.swimming.ca

National Swimming Schools

YMCA
YMCA of the USA
101 N Wacker Drive
Chicago, IL 60606
800-872-9622
www.ymca.net

Swimming Equipment Manufacturers

AQUA SPHERE
2340 Cousteau Court
Vista, CA 92081
800-775-3483
www.aquasphereswim.com/us/

SPEEDO
888-477-3336
www.speedo.com

Swimming Adventure Holidays

SWIMTREK
63 Lansdowne Place
Brighton and Hove
BN3 1FL
Tel: +44 (0)1273 739713

Open-water Swimming

UNITED STATES OPEN WATER SWIMMING
ASSOCIATION (OWSA)
www.usopenwater.org

THE WATER IS OPEN
www.thewaterisopen.com/

Iconic Open-water Swim Organisers

ENGLISH CHANNEL
Channel Swimming and Piloting Federation
www.channelswimming.net

Channel Swimming Association
www.channelswimmingassociation.com

SOLENT
Hants Fish, Hampshire County Council
http://tinyurl.com/yl6p2ju

GIBRALTAR STRAITS
The Straits of Gibraltar Swimming Association
www.acneg.com

HELLESPONT
www.swimtrek.com

INDEX

ACKNOWLEDGMENTS

I would like to thank the team for their fantastic support and guidance in producing this book. Very special thanks go to Jenny Wheatley for agreeing to put up with me for a second time and offering her invaluable knowledge and insight on all aspects of the book, and to Louise Leffler for her outstanding work in the design. Thanks also to Leila Martyn for making the book a reality and her continued support in all areas of my work.

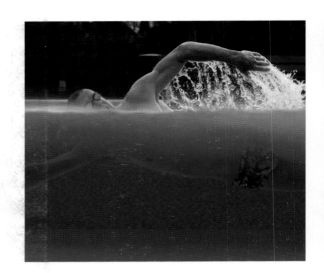

Special thanks go to Eddie Jacob for his awesome photography. Eddie has captured the excitement, fun, and challenge of swimming like no one else could.

Open water photography was shot at Liquid Leisure (Datchet), the River Thames (Marlow), and Brighton. Swimming pool photography was shot at Tooting Bec Lido, Hampton Open Air Pool and The Park Club, East Acton.

I would like to thank Speedo for continuing to support my work and for providing the wonderful swimwear and clothing for this book.

Thanks to my models who undressed and braved the cold: George Whyte (my dad and the inspiration for my swimming career), Steve Whyte (my brother, Channel swimmer and all-around good guy), Nuha Mitchell (mother-in-law, friend, and convert to *Get Fit Not Fat*), Laura Wheatley (thanks also for her support in editing the manuscript), Raquel Meseguer and Rosie Edwards (both braved the very cold waters of Tooting Bec Lido with a smile on their faces), Monjana Fyfe (and bump!), and Mat Wilson and his beautiful daughter Ruby (luckily she doesn't look like her father!).

Most important of all are my girls: Penny, my wife, and my daughters, Maya and Elise, for modeling and being the love of my life.